The Senior Sleep Solution:

A Guide to Improving Sleep in Later Life

Kathy N. Johnson, PhD, CMC

James H. Johnson, PhD

Lily Sarafan, MS

ISBN 978-0-9857236-2-0

OTHER BOOKS BY THE AUTHORS

Happy to 102: The Best Kept Secrets to a Long and Happy Life

The Handbook of Live-in Care: A Guide for Caregivers

From Hospital to Home Care: A Step by Step Guide to Providing Care to Patients Post Hospitalization

Comfort Foods Cookbook: A Healthy Twist on Classic Favorites

The Five Senses: A Sensible Guide to Sensory Loss

Mind Over Gray Matter: A New Approach to Dementia Care

ACKNOWLEDGMENTS

We dedicate this book to the millions of caregivers whose tireless efforts ensure that the loved ones they care for can enjoy a peaceful night's rest.

TABLE OF CONTENTS

INTRODUCTION: SLEEP AND AGING

"It is a common experience that a problem difficult at night is resolved in the morning after the committee of sleep has worked on it." – John Steinbeck

Changes in our sleep patterns are often a normal part of aging—most seniors become sleepy earlier in the evening, tend to have a harder time falling and staying asleep than they did in their younger years and spend less overall time in deep sleep. Waking up tired every day or experiencing highly fragmented sleep every night, however, is not part of the typical aging process. It is important for older adults and the people caring for older adults to be aware of how and why sleep patterns may change with age so that they can spot and remedy disruptions to improve overall quality of life.

Sleeping well is important to our physical and mental wellbeing at every age. Older adults who don't sleep well are more likely to suffer from depression, attention and memory problems, excessive daytime sleepiness and nighttime falls. If you are the primary caregiver for an older adult experiencing sleep problems, it is likely that your sleep will also be disturbed, negatively impacting your health and ability to provide the highest quality of care for your loved one.

If you notice that your loved one is excessively tired during the day, wakes frequently in the night or reports poor sleep quality, there are many possible explanations and solutions. Among the reasons why your loved one may not be sleeping well is the fact that as we age we tend to produce less melatonin, the hormone that promotes sleep, resulting in fragmented sleep. Older adults may also be more sensitive to changes in the environment, such as noise. The prevalence of many sleep disorders, such as insomnia, sleep apnea and restless legs syndrome, also tends to increase with age. Sleep disturbance among seniors can also be attributed to physical and psychiatric health problems and the medications used to treat them. Because some of the underlying conditions that result in sleep problems can have serious health consequences, it can be extremely beneficial to know how to identify changes in your loved one's sleep pattern and communicate them in an educated manner to his or her physician.

This book can help you make informed decisions regarding the care of your loved one. It is divided into three sections. The first section will explain the science of sleep, providing you with working knowledge of what happens during sleep and why we sleep, as well as familiarizing you with terms that you may hear associated with sleep. The second section will address some of the most common barriers to sleep as we age, arming you with the tools to identify warning signs early on in a loved one. Finally, the third section will provide tips for helping your loved one re-establish a restful sleep pattern. The appendices will address the consequences of sleep disturbances in primary caregivers of elderly adults experiencing sleep problems and offer educational print and online resources for additional support and information.

When the root of your loved one's sleep problems is identified and treated, either medically or through simple lifestyle adjustments, his or her quality of sleep (and yours) can be restored. Healthy sleep is vital to overall wellbeing and quality of life and can be achieved at any age.

CHAPTER 1: WHAT IS SLEEP?

"What is it like to fall asleep? What happens? Where do we go?
Why don't we remember? Since childhood, most of us have wondered
about the mystery of sleep." – Henry Reed

It's 10:30 PM and 79-year-old Robert, who stayed up late
watching a football game, is very tired. Yawning, he trades his
jeans and t-shirt for his favorite pair of pajamas and crawls into
bed. His wife, Gina, stirs but doesn't wake up.

Robert quickly finds himself drifting off. Imagining he is falling
through the air, his body jerks awake for a brief period, but he is
soon drowsy again. Finally falling asleep, Robert is no longer aware
of his surroundings. His heart and breathing rates have slowed.

Within half an hour, Robert is deeply asleep. His muscles are
completely relaxed and his breathing rate has slowed even more.
After about an hour and a half, his heart and respiration rates
speed up. His eyes move back and forth quickly under his closed
eyelids. Although his muscles are still deeply relaxed, almost
paralyzed in fact, his brain activity spikes - Robert is dreaming
about going to a college football game with his adult son. The
dream lasts for a little over ten minutes and then Robert shifts
back into a deeper level of sleep. Over the next six to eight hours,
he will repeat this cycle four to five times.

In the morning, Robert will awaken refreshed and in a good
mood. He will have little, if any, memory of what happened to
his body and brain while he was sleeping.

Melatonin

Robert's body actually started preparing for sleep when the sun went down, but he ignored those signals in order to stay up and watch the football game. When his eyes detected darkness, the pineal gland in his brain was triggered to secrete a hormone called melatonin. Often called the "sleep hormone," melatonin causes drowsiness and a decrease in body temperature, which prepare the body to fall asleep.

Melatonin is derived from the neurotransmitter serotonin. Many researchers attribute mental illnesses like depression and anxiety to a serotonin deficiency. Thus, they speculate that one reason some people who are depressed or anxious have trouble falling asleep is that their brains cannot produce the melatonin needed to prepare their bodies for sleep.

The body's production of melatonin decreases with age, which can make it more difficult for seniors to fall and stay asleep.

Brain Waves

To best understand the sleeping brain, we must first look at the waking brain. When a healthy adult is connected to an electroencephalogram (EEG), a device that measures brain waves, the machine will show high levels of activity. Depending on your state of consciousness, the EEG will show different types of waves, including alpha, beta, gamma, delta and theta waves.

Gamma waves have the highest frequency and are associated with good feelings, peak performance and very high levels of cognitive functioning.

Beta waves indicate that the brain is awake and alert. If beta activity starts to fall off, you may notice mood swings, energy levels and a decreased ability to concentrate. Some scientists believe that there is a link between mental illnesses, such as depression, and diminished beta wave activity.

Like beta waves, alpha waves indicate that a person is awake, but in this case, the brain is relaxed and relatively unable to take in or process new information. If you're calm and a little sleepy, you might also show a few theta brain waves. Theta waves signal a small continuum of consciousness ranging from deep relaxation to light sleep. Interestingly, if you look at the EEG of a person who has been hypnotized, you will see multiple theta waves; the higher the concentration, the more impressionable the person will be. Delta waves, the slowest brain waves, do not occur until the deeper stages of sleep.

The Sleeping Brain

When you are awake and alert, an EEG will record mainly gamma and beta waves. As the sun sets and evening falls, you still have many active beta waves, but your alpha waves, the waves that signal relaxation, will also start to populate the EEG. When you prepare for bed and crawl under your covers, the ratio of beta to alpha waves reverses in favor of alpha waves.

The process of sleeping is marked by cycles of activity in the brain that can be divided into five stages. Within 30 minutes of lying down to go to bed, most of us slip into Stage 1 of the sleep cycle. The time it takes you to enter Stage 1 sleep after closing your eyes in bed is called "sleep latency." We will discuss this further in later chapters.

Stage 1 Sleep

As your brain shifts from pre-sleep into the formal sleep cycle, you enter a relatively light stage of rest; stage 1 is a transitional period between being awake and being asleep. An EEG would show multiple alpha and theta waves. If you were awakened during this stage by the phone ringing or by a family member coming into your room, you probably wouldn't realize that you had been asleep at all.

It is in this state that vivid hallucinations, called "hypnagogic hallucinations", may occur (e.g., you hear a voice calling your name or you feel the sensation of falling). These hallucinations can be very frightening, but they pass quickly and we often do not remember them in the morning.

Another event that can occur during this stage of pre-sleep is called the "myoclonic jerk", where the muscles contract or jerk suddenly. Again, this can be a startling experience, but is usually not disruptive enough to prevent us from progressing through the sleep cycle.

You will remain in this initial stage of sleep anywhere from five to ten minutes. Most of us only experience two episodes of Stage 1 sleep each night—the first when we fall asleep and the second when we wake up in the morning.

Stage 2 Sleep

As you move into Stage 2 of sleep, an EEG would start to show rapid, rhythmic brain wave activity known as sleep spindles. No one is completely sure why these sleep spindles occur, but recent research suggests that they may enhance our ability to learn.

During Stage 2 sleep, your body temperature decreases, your heart and respiration rates slow, and overall, your energy is preserved. The brain disengages from the environment so there is a decreased response to outside stimuli. Thus, if you are awakened suddenly during this deeper stage of the sleep cycle, you might feel confused and disoriented for a few seconds.

Stage 2 of the sleep cycle lasts about 20 minutes.

Stage 3 Sleep
Like Stage 1, Stage 3 of the sleep cycle is a transitional stage to deeper sleep. An EEG would start to reflect delta waves, slow waves, which are usually associated with the deepest stages of sleep. In fact, another term for deep sleep is slow-wave sleep (SWS). When more than 50 percent of brain waves are delta waves, you move to Stage 4 of the sleep cycle.

Stage 4 Sleep
Stage 4 is the deepest level of sleep you will experience. An EEG of your brain in this stage of the sleep cycle would be marked mainly by delta waves. Scientists believe that it is during delta wave sleep that your body is restoring itself from wear and tear and resetting any internal clocks that have been disrupted. Delta waves also signal the release of growth hormones meaning that the number of times we enter this stage of sleep may actually make a difference in our physique.

In this stage, your blood pressure and your breathing rate decrease even more, and your muscles become completely relaxed.

Because you are deeply unconscious, you might not arouse in time to tend to your body's needs; bedwetting and sleepwalking tend to occur at the end of Stage 4.

The first time your body reaches Stage 4 sleep during the night, it usually remains in that stage for about an hour. Afterwards, as additional sleep cycles occur, the body usually stays in Stage 3 and Stage 4 sleep for about five to 15 minutes each.

Stage 5 (REM Sleep)

The final stage of the sleep cycle is named "REM" sleep for rapid eye movement because if you look at a person in REM sleep, you can see his or her eyes move quickly back and forth under the closed lids.

Interestingly, the body does not enter Stage 5 sleep directly from Stage 4. Instead, you may go through the earlier stages a few times before entering REM. So, the actual sleep cycle might look something like this:

1→2→3→4→3→2→REM→ (starting a new cycle)
2→3→4→3→2→REM

Most dreaming occurs during REM sleep. An EEG during this stage would closely resemble one recorded during wakefulness. Similarly, your body reflects this heightened activity as eye movements, heart rate and respiration increase. Your muscles, however, are paralyzed during this stage of sleep. Researchers believe this may be a self-protective mechanism so that you don't hurt yourself trying to act out your dreams. If you've ever had a nightmare that someone or something was chasing you but you couldn't move, it's because of this sleep paralysis. Once you are aroused from REM sleep or slip into the next stage of the sleep cycle, your muscles will begin to function normally once again.

You will usually reach REM sleep about 90 minutes after you first fall asleep. The initial period of REM sleep may last about 10 minutes with each recurring stage increasing up to a period of one hour.

To achieve a healthy amount of rest, a person needs to go through four or five complete sleep cycles each night.

Waking Up

In the morning, we may be awakened by a loud noise, like an alarm clock going off or the beeping of the garbage truck as it backs into the driveway. Sometimes the body has kept the same sleep schedule for so long that the brain has been conditioned to return to a waking state at a certain time. In general, two hormones play major roles in the way we wake up.

Melatonin, the "sleep hormone" is triggered by darkness, but inhibited by light. As the sun shines through the window and into your room, receptors in your eyes signal the pineal gland to stop secreting melatonin. This diminishes drowsiness and raises your body temperature slightly, getting you ready to start the day.

About half an hour after waking up, 70 percent of people receive a cortisol boost, a phenomenon scientists have coined the **"Cortisol Awakening Response"** (CAR). The reason for this sudden surge of cortisol is not well understood, but may have something to do with shaking off the last vestiges of sleep and preparing for the stressors that the day will bring.

The Aging Brain Asleep

As we will discuss in more detail in subsequent chapters, older adults tend to experience lighter, more fragmented sleep with less overall time spent in deep sleep. Thus, a senior may fall asleep and reach Stage 2 of the sleep cycle, but wake up before he or she can reach deep sleep or REM sleep. This pattern may occur several times each night.

Many doctors believe that these sleep problems are not necessarily due to aging itself, but rather to the many different health problems seniors experience including reactions to medications, aches and pains, sleep apnea and depression. When these conditions are identified and treated, most seniors report that the quality of their sleep improves.

Now that you've learned the basics behind the different stages of sleep and what happens to the body and brain during each stage, you may be wondering why we need to sleep at all. The next chapter will address the many ways the body and brain repair themselves while we sleep as well as the consequences of getting too little sleep.

CHAPTER 2: WHY DO WE SLEEP?

"Sleep is the golden chain that ties health and our bodies together."
– Thomas Dekker

Why do we sleep? In spite of decades of research, scientists still
aren't exactly sure how to answer this question. From a strictly
evolutionary standpoint, it seems that organisms should have
adapted beyond a need for sleep, as the process is not conducive
to survival: sleep is a time when we are defenseless and vulnerable
to predators and rather unproductive. But, that every other
living creature on the earth also enters a sleeplike state each day
underscores the importance of this process for survival.

In fact, sleep deprivation has significant negative effects on
the body and mind. Studies have shown that after 48 hours
of wakefulness, people begin to experience hallucinations,
decreased immune response, impaired memory and cognitive
processes, increased sensitivity to pain and increased suggestibility.
As a result, Amnesty International decrees sleep deprivation
a Cruel, Inhuman and Degrading (CID) practice outlawed
under both U.S. and international law.

People who do not obtain the amount of sleep their bodies require
tend to exhibit slow reflexes, poor decision making skills, memory
impairments and irritability. Some studies suggest that driving
while sleep-deprived is as dangerous as driving while intoxicated.

If sleep deprivation continues beyond a few days, it can lead to an
even more deadly outcome than impaired driving. In the 1980s,
researchers at the University of Chicago investigated the effects
of sleep deprivation on rats. They prevented the rodents from

sleeping, though they continued to provide food, water and other necessities. Within two weeks, all of the rats were dead. Despite extensive necropsies, the research team found no organ or tissue damage; thus, the only reason they could offer for the deaths was exhaustion given the sheer lack of sleep.

A handful of humans have also died from sleep deprivation. There is a rare genetic condition, which has been identified in only 40 families throughout the world, called fatal familial insomnia (FFI). Symptoms usually appear in middle age and manifest as disruptions in the ability to nap. Soon, however, the person has trouble falling asleep at night. Sleep comes later and later each night, until finally it does not come at all. Anxiety, hallucinations, delirium and confusion result. The disease always ends in death, usually within about a year of symptom onset. Similar to the outcome of the University of Chicago study, scientists hypothesize a relationship between the complete lack of sleep and death.

There is no question that humans do need sleep. Lack of sleep impacts our health, safety and longevity. We're just not sure why we need it.

Possible Functions of Sleep

There are multiple theories designed to explain why we sleep. Two theories we will address here focus on the processes of restoration and learning. During sleep, our bodies repair cell damage experienced during the day and our brains encode information in the form of memories.

Repairing the Body. We can often be hard on our bodies during the day. Some of the damages we inflict are intentional and beneficial. Resistance training, for instance, works because contracting a muscle against an external force causes miniscule tears in the muscle. As the body heals those tears, the muscle becomes stronger and larger.

Other damage is not so beneficial. Free radicals are the by-products of our metabolism at work. Over time, too many free radicals may harm our tissues. Some researchers even attest to a correlation between the concentration of free radicals in our bodies and the development of cancer, heart disease, stroke and even the aging process itself.

With all the activity that occurs during the day, sleep provides an opportunity to repair and rejuvenate damaged cells. One piece of evidence that supports this theory is the fact that the body secretes growth hormone primarily, or sometimes solely, during the sleep cycle (see Stage 4, page 7). In addition, muscle growth, tissue repair and protein synthesis, the major restorative functions of the body, occur during sleep. Further evidence suggests that sleep is necessary for optimal immune function. Studies have shown that wounds on rats are slower to heal if the rats are sleep-deprived. Though evidence in the human immune system is inconclusive, researchers continue to investigate the possibility.

Most of the activity that seems aimed at repairing the body happens during deep sleep, usually during Stage 4.

Learning and Memory. Research suggests that sleep, particularly REM sleep, is necessary for learning and memory. It allows the brain to process, organize and store what was learned during the day. Consolidating memory is essential for learning new information. Studies that measure brain activity on subjects both when they are awake and when they are asleep have found that, during REM sleep, the neurons in the brain will repeat patterns of firing that occurred when the subjects were awake and learning a new task.

If the brain does use the time spent during REM sleep to process and solidify memories, this could explain why dreams often feel so real and familiar—they may contain elements of the very things we have just seen, learned or experienced. It could also explain why people who are unable to sleep exhibit increased forgetfulness. Some researchers believe that the hallucinations that begin to occur after about two days without sleep are the brain's desperate attempts to try to process and store memories while awake.

Sleep may also play a role in regulating mood and attention, both of which are important to learning ability. A study conducted at the University of California – Berkeley, examined the potential link between sleep and emotion regulation efficacy. Subjects were assigned to a sleep group or a wakeful group. Brain scans were obtained using functional magnetic resonance imaging (fMRI) while each participant looked through 150 emotionally intense photographs. Those in the sleep group then slept for eight hours while those in the wakeful group were instructed not to sleep. Twelve hours after the initial photo viewing sessions, the subjects repeated the task.

Those who had slept exhibited a decrease in activity in the amygdala (the part of the brain thought to play a role in emotional learning) during viewing. The subjects who had stayed awake, however, showed more activity than they had initially. When researchers interviewed the subjects, they found that members of the group that slept were more likely to report that the pictures were "neutral," while members of the group that stayed awake reported finding the pictures as emotionally intense as they had the first time they viewed them. Thus, it seemed that sleep rejuvenated the individuals' abilities to regulate emotion. It appears that the old adage, "Just sleep on it and you'll feel better," may have a basis in neurobiology.

Just as the body may clear free radicals during sleep, the brain may be doing some housekeeping as well. During our waking hours, we pick up all sorts of information consciously and unconsciously. Some of it is vital or at least important (e.g., survival skills, lessons that you will be expected to remember for a test), but most of it is either trivial or already known (e.g., your spouse's name, how to defrost a frozen dinner). Researchers have speculated that during REM sleep, the brain might rid itself of redundant information or unneeded connections between neurons.

Final Answers?

Despite decades of research, the question of why we sleep still has no definitive answer. Educated guesses, as well as experiments and observations, have given researchers clues about what might be going on in the body and the brain during sleep. It is fairly obvious, for instance, that the body uses the downtime to restore and repair itself, but we cannot yet explain the exact process by which this repair occurs. We also cannot point to any one organ that suffers obvious damage in people or animals that die from sleep deprivation.

Similarly, we can tell from looking at brain scans that the brain is almost as active in REM sleep as it is when it is awake. Researchers believe this has significance for both cognition (the way we think) and mood (the way we feel), but again they cannot explain exactly how the brain solidifies important memories, takes the edge off traumatic memories and disposes of duplicate or unnecessary memories.

When it comes to the reasons that we need sleep, the brain and the body are still keeping us in the dark.

While our need for sleep does not change as we age, the quality of our sleep may change. The next chapter looks at the sleep cycle at different life stages.

CHAPTER 3: SLEEP CYCLES AT DIFFERENT LIFE STAGES

"The amount of sleep required by the average person is five minutes more." – *Wilson Mizener*

Carla, age 70, has been having a hard time getting to sleep at night. Because she has difficulty breathing, she needs to remain fairly upright and use supplemental oxygen while sleeping.

Carla lies down around 9:00 PM but quickly becomes anxious as her mind races with various worries: her financial problems and the repairs her home needs before winter. She wishes she had family members living close by who could help. Eventually, she becomes too tired to keep her eyes open and falls asleep around 1:00 AM. She wakes up again at 5:00 AM sharp as she has done every day for the past 50 years. Sometimes she is so tired that she takes short naps throughout the day.

Carla's friends tell her that she shouldn't worry and that older people simply don't need as much sleep as younger people. Are they right?

Sleep Requirements as We Age

From infancy through the first year of life, we need 16 to 20 hours of sleep every day. Of course, as every exhausted parent of a newborn could tell you, babies don't get all their sleep in one big chunk. Instead they rest for a few hours, wake up to nurse or to interact with caregivers, and then fall back to sleep for another few hours.

As an infant grows to be a toddler, we see changes in the amount of sleep required and the period over which sleep occurs. Between the ages of one and four, children generally require 11 to 12 hours of sleep. This often comes in a large block of sleep at night and a nap or two during the day. From the age of four years through adolescence, most children drop the nap and sleep fewer hours each night. Contrary to popular belief, older adults need about the same amount of sleep as younger adults—generally seven to nine hours per night.

"But I can get by on less than that!" you may be saying. Perhaps. The University of California, San Francisco, has discovered a gene that allows people to function on fewer than six hours of sleep per night, but only three percent of the population carries this gene. If you believe that you are actually at optimal performance with just a few hours of sleep, consider making an appointment at a sleep clinic to have this formally assessed.

Quality of Sleep as We Age

Sleep disturbances can begin as early as age 11. In fact, 7 out of 10 young and middle-aged adults experience at least occasional problems getting to sleep and staying asleep. Fifty percent of people over the age of 65 report frequent sleeping problems.

When they do fall asleep, seniors are likely to sleep lightly and for a short time span before waking again. This means that older adults may have trouble reaching deep sleep and REM sleep, the sleep stage vital to healing and memory.

Are the Elderly Chronically Sleep-Deprived?

Some studies have suggested that the elderly do not need as much sleep as their counterparts in young adulthood and middle age. One study, conducted by Harvard Medical School and the Brigham and Women's Hospital compared the sleep quality of 35 subjects between the ages of 18 and 32 to a group of 18 subjects between the ages of 60 and 75. When researchers inquired about subjects' sleep, they found that the younger group slept for an average of nine hours while the older group only slept for an average of 7.5 hours. This led researchers to conclude that seniors require 1.5 fewer hours of sleep per night than their younger counterparts. However, just because seniors may sleep less doesn't mean they actually need less sleep.

In a study conducted at the University of California–San Diego researchers monitored a younger group (average age of 27) and an older group (average age of 68) of participants for two nights in a sleep laboratory. On the second day of the study, researchers gave each subject a list of words to memorize. The older subjects' ability to memorize the list was strongly linked to the amount of sleep they had the night before. Those who had slept for fewer hours remembered fewer words. Though sleep was also correlated with performance for the younger group, the relationship was not as strong. These researchers also concluded that senior citizens require several continuous hours of sleep. Dr. Sean Drummond, the head of the research team, explained that a solid chunk of sleep allows the brain to act as a sponge when it comes to learning new material. Short naps throughout the day or periods of sleeping and waking at night do not provide the restorative sleep that the body requires.

The next chapter will focus on one of the most common barriers to quality sleep: occasional insomnia.

CHAPTER 4: COMMON CAUSES OF OCCASIONAL INSOMNIA

"But I have promises to keep, and miles to go before I sleep…"
– Robert Frost

Seven out of ten adults report occasional problems falling and staying asleep. Though these disruptions are not pleasant, they usually pass pretty quickly, sometimes after only one night. This chapter looks at some of the reasons why occasional insomnia may occur and offers suggestions for correcting these problems.

Noise

One of the running jokes in the 1992 movie, *My Cousin Vinny*, is attorney Vinny Gambini's fruitless efforts to find a place in the Southern countryside where he can get a good night's sleep without being awakened by strange noises. After being woken up by a train, a herd of farm animals, an owl and finally a thunderstorm, Vinny can hardly stay awake to defend his clients. At last, he allows himself to be taken into custody on a contempt of court charge. Though there is a riot in the prison that night, the seasoned New York native sleeps like a baby.

Across age groups, noise is cited as one of the chief causes of occasional insomnia. Whether it's loud housemates, the noise from the television or radio, or a loudly snoring partner, the brain can become distracted by processing sounds rather than preparing for sleep.

If disruptive noise is contributing to sleep problems for your loved one, there are several things that you can try.

Ban the TV and other electronics from the bedroom. It's practically impossible to get quality sleep with the television, radio, mp3 player, etc. blaring in the background. Even if your loved one is used to having the TV playing and thinks he or she can sleep well with it on, the truth of the matter is that he or she is probably not getting a good night's rest. In fact, chances are that your loved one is waking up briefly dozens of times a night as certain words or songs catch his or her ear. Give your loved one's body and brain a break and gently wean him or her off of falling asleep with the television or music in the background.

Discuss excessive noise with neighbors. Some neighbors are considerate about not making noise after a certain time in the evening, but others may not be so respectful. Consider visiting your loved one's neighbors in the mid-afternoon to explain the problem, if one exists, and look for win-win scenarios. If your loved one shares a wall (e.g. townhouses) perhaps the neighbor could put up soundproof mats or pillows on the wall. You may also discuss setting quiet hours for the weekdays and weekends.

One man, Ray, an 83-year-old widower who lived in a rural area, came up with a unique solution to a noise problem. Ray's neighbor raised cattle and parked loaded trailers in his driveway overnight. The problem was that the cows milled around in the metal trailer and mooed to each other all night, disturbing Ray's sleep. He tried to talk this problem over with his neighbor, but found him to be quite unsympathetic. "Hey, it's my driveway," the neighbor said, "and they don't bother me."

The next time the trailer appeared in the neighbor's driveway, Ray waited until a little after 1:00 AM and then telephoned the neighbor. When the sleepy man answered the phone, Ray said,

"I just wanted to let you know that your cows are doing fine. I'll call you with another update in about an hour."

The neighbor hastily moved the trailer to the back of his property and Ray was never bothered by noisy cows again. While this exchange is not typical, it highlights the importance of communicating needs with neighbors or housemates to ensure that the environment is not needlessly contributing to your loved one's sleep problems.

Complain. If your loved one lives in an apartment complex, notify the apartment managers if his or her neighbors are excessively noisy at night. Most communities have noise ordinances. You can call the police if the neighbors are in violation of any of these statutes.

Put thick curtains over the windows. Thick curtains not only block unwanted light from coming in the room, but they can also muffle outside sounds. Plus, they are an elegant solution because they can add to the ambience of your loved one's bedroom.

Purchase a white noise machine. A white noise machine plays gentle static or nature sounds like waves or rain. Focusing on these sounds can block out other, more annoying noises. A fan can also create white noise, and many people find it soothing to sleep with air blowing over them.

Try a sleep mask and/or ear plugs. Some sleep masks are designed so that they cover both the eyes and ears. You might also consider buying a pair of earplugs designed to filter out excess noise at night. You may find that your loved one is not comfortable sleeping with masks or earplugs, but since they typically don't cost very much, it's well worth your money and your loved one's health to give them a try.

Move to a new location. If you've exhausted all possible strategies, your loved one may consider finding a new home in a quieter neighborhood.

Sandra, age 77, was happy to find an apartment next to a street with service stations, strip malls and a couple of large grocery stores. What she hadn't taken into account was the traffic on the street both day and night. Sandra's apartment was also less than a mile away from the nearest hospital, so she was often awakened by sirens at night. She tried several of the suggestions listed above, but found that the noise still prevented her from sleeping well. When her lease was over, she moved to an apartment complex in a residential area away from the hustle and bustle.

Pain

Whether it's a passing headache or chronic, longstanding discomfort, such as the inflammation from arthritis, pain can interfere with the relaxation response that leads to sleep. It's difficult to relax when the mind is focused on a throbbing head, leg or arm. Common types of pain that make sleep difficult include:

- Headache (migraine or tension)
- Muscle aches due to over-exertion
- Arthritis—inflammation of the joints
- Heart burn and other stomach pains
- Lower back pain
- Scrapes, cuts, bruises and other injuries
- Foot pain due to bone spurs, ingrown toenails, etc.

There are several steps you can take if pain is keeping your loved one from getting his or her beauty sleep.

Check with a doctor. If your loved one is experiencing chronic pain, sudden, acute pain, or difficulty walking after a fall or other injury, see a doctor right away. A doctor can assess the root of the pain and suggest ways to manage discomfort, although pain is not always easily treated. If this is the case, ask your loved one's doctor for a referral to a pain clinic where a team of medical professionals can offer further suggestions and diagnoses.

Apply heat. Warm showers and baths or a warm washcloth or heating pad applied to the sore area can relax tense, aching muscles and encourage sleep. If a heating pad is used, avoid turning it up to the highest setting as it can burn your loved one's skin and cause even more pain. Be sure to unplug the heating pad once your loved one is done using it to ensure his or her safety.

Apply cold. If the pain is due to inflammation, a cool compress or ice wrapped in a washcloth may be exactly what is needed. The cold helps to reduce the swelling and numb the pain.

Consider medications. Most types of pain can be relieved with the recommended doses of over-the-counter analgesics (pain relievers). If your loved one is taking other medications or if he or she has numerous health problems, check with his or her doctor or pharmacist before introducing new medications. For severe pain, doctors may prescribe stronger painkillers. Using these as directed will usually ease the pain and relax your loved one enough for him or her to fall asleep.

Alcohol

Many people will consume a few beers or glasses of wine to help them relax and fall asleep. Initially, this may seem like an ideal solution; alcohol is a depressant and therefore reduces the amount of time it takes to fall asleep.

Unfortunately, alcohol also severely compromises the quality of sleep by disturbing the second half of the sleep cycle. It may cause your loved one to sleep fitfully, awaken during REM sleep as well as make it hard for him or her to fall back asleep.

Waking up during REM sleep can have significant consequences. First, your loved one may retain vivid memories of his or her dreams, which can be bizarre or even frightening.

Second, because REM sleep is the stage of the sleep cycle during which we categorize and solidify memories your loved one may experience cognitive problems, such as memory impairments, with consistent use of alcohol.

In addition, people who consume alcohol prior to bedtime tend to awaken multiple times during the night. As a result, they often report daytime sleepiness and increased levels of fatigue.

Alcohol used before bedtime can pose a special risk to seniors, as they are more vulnerable to its effects than their younger counterparts. Seniors who awaken during the REM cycle are also at risk of getting out of bed and falling due to confusion and/or intoxication.

If your loved one has been using alcohol to fall asleep at night consider the following alternatives:

Avoid consuming alcohol at least two hours prior to bedtime. Suggest that your loved one switch to a non-alcoholic, caffeine-free drink instead.

Limit alcohol intake earlier in the evening. Try to ensure that your loved one drinks no more than one or two alcoholic beverages.

Get help if needed. If cutting back on alcohol is a problem for your loved one, talk to his or her doctor and/or to a licensed mental health professional. They can assess your loved one's drinking habits and help him or her develop a plan to reduce or stop drinking if necessary.

Suggest that your loved one wear a personal medical alarm. If your loved one lives alone, wearing a personal medical alarm will allow him or her to summon help quickly in the event of a fall or other emergency. It is especially important for your loved one to wear an alarm if he or she has suffered falls in the past due to alcohol consumption.

Caffeine

Caffeine is a plant product found in coffee, tea, cocoa, chocolate, some soft drinks and some prescription and over-the-counter medications. It stimulates the central nervous system and increases alertness. The National Sleep Foundation refers to caffeine as "the most popular drug in the world."

Caffeine meets no nutritional need, but researchers say there is probably no harm in moderate intake (about three cups of coffee per day).

One problem with caffeine and sleep is that caffeine has a half-life of about six hours. That means that if you drink two cups of coffee at 3:00 PM, half of the caffeine you consume will still be in your body at 9:00 PM. People over the age of 65 may take even longer to metabolize caffeine.

Because it is a stimulant, caffeine can wreak havoc on your loved one's sleep schedule. Not only does it block adenosine, a sleep-inducing chemical in the brain, but it can also increase sleep latency, cause frequent awakenings, and reduce total sleep time and time spent in deep sleep.

Many people wake up from a caffeine-disturbed sleep only to grab another cup of coffee or a soft drink to give them the caffeine boost they feel they need to start the day and make up for lack of restful sleep. This behavior can create a vicious cycle of caffeine-disturbed sleep.

Some over-the-counter medications, including pain relievers like Excedrin, use caffeine as an ingredient. Thus, it's important to discuss ingredients and side effects of all medications with your loved one's doctor or pharmacist.

If your loved one is having difficulty sleeping due to caffeine usage, try the following suggestions:

Check medications for the presence of caffeine. If you are not sure what to look for on the labels, talk to a doctor or pharmacist. The doctor may be able to prescribe your loved one a similar medication that does not contain caffeine.

Avoid caffeine after 12:00 PM. If your loved one drinks or eats caffeinated products in the afternoon, the caffeine will still be lingering in his or her system when it's time to rest in the evening; try giving your loved one a decaffeinated cup of coffee or green tea. It's possible he or she may not even notice the difference and you can start replacing caffeinated beverages with decaffeinated beverages instead.

Expect withdrawal symptoms. If your loved one cuts back on caffeine or stops using it altogether, he or she may experience headaches, difficulty concentrating and feelings of irritability or depression. These symptoms are usually mild, but if they become disruptive, consult with a physician.

Normal Anxiety/Worry

For some of us, lying down in bed seems to trigger the brain to focus on life events or circumstances that are causing stress or concern. Some of the most common worries that older adults have relate to health, money and aging. Thinking about upsetting topics keeps the body tense and makes it harder for your loved one to relax and fall asleep.

Some people get into a vicious cycle when it comes to worry and sleep. On the one hand, they can't fall asleep because they're stressed out. On the other hand, they know they need a good night's sleep to function at their highest level the next day. Soon, the stress and the frustration of not being able to sleep are almost as disruptive as the original stressor. If anxious thoughts or worries are keeping your loved one awake, you can try several possible solutions:

Suggest getting up for a while. Average sleep latency is 20 to 30 minutes after going to bed. If your loved one is still tossing and turning after half an hour, encourage him or her to get up and engage in a quiet, distracting activity like reading, working on a crossword puzzle, or listening to soft music until he or she feels ready to sleep.

Offer a journal. Encourage your loved one to express his or her worries on paper. That way, your loved one has a chance to address and release them before going to bed.

Practice simple relaxation techniques. One of the easiest methods is progressive muscle relaxation (PMR). Have your loved one sit or lie down in a comfortable position. Then, starting with the toes and feet, coach your loved one to clench and relax each muscle group (calves, hips, etc.). Some people also find meditating or listening to guided-visualization calming.

Give your loved one a reality check. If your loved one is worried about losing sleep, remind him or her that as long as he or she sleeps seven to nine hours on most nights, an occasional wakeful night won't do any harm. The worst-case scenario is that he or she will feel a little tired and grumpy the next day. Coming to this realization may help your loved one restructure his or her stress-provoking cognitions around the topic of sleep.

Insomnia and Senior Citizens

Older adults tend to sleep lightly and thus may be easily disturbed by changes in the environment, such as noise. They are also more sensitive to the effects of alcohol, caffeine and other drugs and medications. Pain and psychological stress are also common causes of insomnia in older adults. Because seniors who get up and walk around during the night are vulnerable to falling, which can result in serious injury and hospital admission, if your elderly loved one lives alone with no family close by, it may be a good idea to hire a trained, compassionate caregiver to stay overnight. A caregiver can help your loved one establish a comfortable and relaxing bedtime routine to encourage sleep as well as provide reassurance and supervision if your loved one wakes up confused and disoriented.

A caregiver can also help your loved one avoid naps by staying active and engaged during the day. While a quick catnap probably won't hurt your loved one, any nap that lasts longer than 15 to 30 minutes may throw off his or her sleep cycle and make it difficult to fall asleep at bedtime.

The next chapter will focus on chronic insomnia and other sleep disturbances that result from the progression of Alzheimer's and other forms of dementia.

CHAPTER 5: DEMENTIA

"Caring for an Alzheimer's patient is a situation that can utterly consume the lives and well-being of the people giving care, just as the disorder consumes its victims." – Leeza Gibbons

As of 2013, around six million individuals throughout North America are living with Alzheimer's disease or another type of dementia. The neurodegenerative changes associated with dementia increase the frequency and severity of sleep disturbances. According to a 2009 study published in *Geriatrics*, 35 percent of people living with dementia in their own or in loved ones' homes experience insomnia while 40 to 70 percent of dementia patients living in nursing facilities experience sleep disturbances.

Insomnias and parasomnias (unwanted experiences during sleep) significantly contribute to the burden on family caregivers (see Appendix A). For this reason, hiring a professional caregiver to provide around-the-clock care is a smart solution and will ensure both the safety of the care recipient and the peace of mind of his or her loved ones.

Sleep and Dementia

The Alzheimer's Association has documented that people with dementia experience longer sleep latencies and wake up more frequently during the night than people who do not have dementia. They also spend less time in REM sleep and deep sleep (Stages 3 and 4). Researchers attribute these sleep issues to the degeneration (irreversible loss of function) of neurons in the brain as dementia progresses. The lack of REM sleep, the time during which memories are processed and solidified, may compound the troubles with learning and memory associated with dementia.

People with dementia also often experience disturbances in the circadian rhythm, or the sleep-wake cycle. What may begin as occasional napping during the day may eventually evolve into a complete disorientation of time. Those with advanced Alzheimer's have difficulty reading and acting upon environmental cues. For most of us, eating dinner, watching the sky grow dark outside, and watching our favorite news program before bed all signal our body and brain to prepare for sleep. For a person with severe dementia, these activities have lost their significance. In fact, researchers have found that among people with advanced dementia, at least 40 percent experience a complete reversal in the sleep-wake cycle—they stay up all night and sleep all day.

Another sleep-associated consequence of dementia is "sundowning." It is most often experienced during the middle stage of Alzheimer's disease and in mixed dementias, where more than one disease process is causing cognitive decline. Patients who experience sundowning exhibit a number of behavioral problems in the evening or while the sun is setting. Symptoms may include increased confusion, agitation and even aggression. Though a specific cause of sundowning has not been scientifically verified, some researchers believe that the destruction of neurons is the most likely culprit. If certain parts of the brain are damaged by illness or injury, it may be difficult or almost impossible to get a full night's sleep. As dementia progresses, it is likely that these parts of the brain, along with many others, become impaired.

Treating Dementia-Related Insomnia and Parasomnias

If your loved one is having trouble falling asleep and staying asleep, or if he or she is suffering from nightmares or other unwanted nighttime events, there are several interventions you can try with him or her:

Introduce a routine. One of the best ways to deal with a reversal of the sleep-wake cycle is to introduce a consistent routine of planned daily activities. Rather than allowing your loved one to nap all day, encourage him or her to participate in household chores, exercise, games and social activities. For instance, morning might consist of personal care such as a shower or a bath and breakfast while afternoons might be spent taking a walk through the local park and a game of dominoes.

Focus evening activities on settling down and getting ready to sleep. You might, for instance, offer your loved one a light meal or snack, help him or her into pajamas or a nightgown, and devise a bedtime ritual like saying a prayer and what you are thankful for, looking at family pictures in a photo album or reading a favorite book. If your loved one's daily routine includes a nap, be sure it is no longer than 30 minutes.

Use reality orientation. During the day, orient your loved one to time. For instance, you might say, "It's ten o'clock in the morning—time for our walk," or "It's two o'clock in the afternoon. That's when *Gilligan's Island* comes on." Be especially sure to let your loved one know when bedtime is approaching. For example, you can say, "In about thirty minutes it will be time for us to go to sleep."

Spend time outdoors. Another way to help your loved one re-establish a normal circadian rhythm is to make sure that he or she spends time outside in the sunlight. Talk to your loved one's doctor or pharmacist before taking him or her outside for extended periods of time. Certain medical conditions and medications can make your loved one more sensitive to the sun's rays, so you may need to shorten your time outside or make sure your loved one protects him or herself by wearing a hat and sunscreen with a high SPF.

Arrange for exercise. Exercise during the day will also help your loved one sleep better at night. Just be sure that the exercise takes place in the morning or early afternoon. Strenuous exercise just before bedtime can actually delay the onset of sleep. One of the best and easiest forms of exercise is simply taking a walk. One study found that most people with early to mid-stage dementia were able to walk at a steady pace for about 30 minutes. Some people with dementia also enjoy swimming, water aerobics, yoga and tai chi.

If your loved one's mobility is limited, start slowly; a five minute walk is better than no activity at all. Even a person in a wheelchair can be encouraged to raise and lower his or her arms, shrug his or her shoulders, do head rolls and even play catch with a large, soft ball. If you're not sure which exercises would be most appropriate for your loved one, talk to his or her doctor.

Pay attention to the environment. If your loved one wakes up at night with bad dreams, take a closer look at his or her surroundings. If the television or radio is on and your loved one wakes up in the middle of the night, he or she may find the noise confusing.

Edna, for instance, an 85-year-old woman with moderate dementia lived next door to her son in an apartment building. Every morning at about 3:15 AM she would knock at his door and say that the police were in her apartment and wouldn't leave. When her son investigated, he found no one else in the apartment.

After these sleep disturbances had been going on for a couple of weeks, Edna's son finally figured out what was going on: Edna kept the television set on when she fell asleep and she typically would wake up early in the morning to use the bathroom. The television show *Cops*, which was often loud and violent, was on at 3:00 AM. Edna heard the noise and didn't realize that the police were on television, not in her apartment. Her son convinced her to turn the TV to a channel that played soft classical music and the problem was resolved.

Treat pain. Many older people have various aches and pains like arthritis, headaches and muscle aches but as dementia progresses, people tend to have difficulty communicating and may not say they are in pain. If you suspect that pain is one of the factors contributing to your loved one's inability to sleep, talk to his or her doctor. The doctor may suggest a low dose of over-the-counter pain medication such as ibuprofen or acetaminophen. If the pain is severe, the doctor may prescribe something stronger like an opioid pain reliever.

Hire a caregiver. If your loved one experiences sundowning or has a reversed sleep-wake cycle, it can take a lot of time and patience to restore normal sleep. Many family caregivers find that the burden is too heavy for one person to handle. Hiring a caregiver to come in at night allows you to rest without worrying that your loved one will get up and injure him or herself while wandering. A caregiver can also give you suggestions on interacting with your loved one in ways that encourage relaxation and sleep.

Dementia Therapeutics

Dementia Therapeutics, part of Home Care Assistance's suite of care options, is a non-pharmacological program that works to slow the progression of dementia. It offers personalized in-home interventions (activities) based on each client's unique needs, abilities, limitations, interests, preferences and histories. The interventions are centered around five areas of cognitive functioning that are most affected by dementia: executive functioning, attention, language, visual-spatial perception and memory. Sensory, coping, social and recreational needs are also addressed.

Dementia Therapeutics is a comprehensive approach and also provides educational resources and support programs for the families. Loved ones are provided with regular updates on the client's progress.

Getting your loved one involved in Dementia Therapeutics serves several purposes. First, working with the interventionist may slow the rate of cognitive decline. Second, visits with the interventionist help establish a regular, healthy routine for your loved one. Finally, the interventionist can teach you more effective ways to interact with your loved one so that you do not become as frustrated by common problems like insomnia.

Caring for a loved one with dementia can be a significant challenge for even the most compassionate and patient caregiver. Trying to do it alone is practically impossible. Hire a professional caregiver, take advantage of programs like Dementia Therapeutics, research adult day care centers in your area and encourage other family members to help as much as they can—if not physically, then at least financially.

The next chapter looks at a common sleep disturbance among travelers of all ages: jet lag. Years ago, when people traveled long distances by ship or by car, jet lag was not a significant problem. Now that airplanes have become the preferred mode of long-distance transportation, more people are experiencing jet lag. Jet lag can be especially harsh on older adults, with more people traveling regularly well into their 80s and 90s. If you are traveling across several time zones with an aging loved one, it's important for you to know how jet lag can affect him or her and how to relieve these symptoms.

CHAPTER 6: JET LAG

"Jet lag is your soul trying to catch up with you after flying."
– Ryan Ross

Marie was born in France. After World War II, she married an American GI and moved to New York with him. They loved each other deeply and raised two daughters and a son. Marie enjoyed New York, but often longed to visit the French village where she had been born. She especially wanted to meet her nieces and nephews. This desire grew even stronger after her husband died unexpectedly, so she started saving to take the trip back to her village.

A year after her husband's death, she had finally saved enough so that she and her oldest daughter could visit France together.

Unfortunately, the beginning of the trip did not go as well as she had anticipated. She was nervous about flying and stayed awake for the entire time the plane was in the air. By the time she and her daughter reached their destination, Marie was exhausted and didn't feel well. She wasn't in the mood for sightseeing.

She told herself that she would be all right after a good night's sleep, but she tossed and turned for hours before sleep finally came. The next morning she was groggy and had an upset stomach. She was pleased when two of her great-nieces came to the hotel to visit her, but she still didn't feel like going out.

After two more unpleasant days, Marie's daughter took her to see a local physician. His assessment was that Marie was experiencing jet lag. He told Marie to spend time each morning sitting in the sunlight, even if she didn't feel like it. Marie followed the doctor's instructions and her symptoms started to improve. By the end of the two-week trip, she felt like herself again. She declared the journey a success, even though she regretted not being able to enjoy the first week as much as she would have liked.

Jet lag is a temporary sleep disruption that some people experience after crossing multiple time zones over a relatively short period of time. Time zones run from north to south, with an hour difference between each division. In the continental United States, for instance, there are four time zones: Pacific, Mountain, Central and Eastern with a total of three hours difference between the Pacific and Eastern zones; if it is 1:00 PM Pacific time, it is 4:00 PM Eastern time.

Jet lag—which got its name because slower modes of travel are not as disruptive to sleep rhythms—occurs when your circadian rhythm is thrown off balance due to changes in environmental cues. If your body expects dark, for instance, but your eyes see light, your brain isn't sure whether it should be asleep or awake.

Jet Lag Symptoms

Symptoms of jet lag can include insomnia, increased sleep latency, early waking, sleepiness during the day, problems with concentration and memory, muscle aches, gastrointestinal problems such as upset stomach or diarrhea and a general sense of feeling off. Though they cause discomfort, most of the symptoms are not life threatening. On the rare occasions when jet lag has been associated with fatal outcomes such as heart attack and stroke, victims were usually older travelers with several pre-existing conditions.

Most people do not experience symptoms of jet lag unless they have crossed at least three time zones. Because people traveling west "gain" time and people traveling east "lose" time, it is usually harder to adapt to traveling east than to traveling west. Those who travel from west to east are more likely to have trouble falling asleep at night and waking up in the morning when they reach their destination. Those who travel from east to west, on the other hand, generally experience early evening sleepiness and wake up in the pre-dawn hours.

Risk Factors for Jet Lag

Risk factors associated with developing jet lag include:
- Crossing a large number of time zones
- Flying east
- Flying frequently
- Advanced age

Jet Lag Remedies

Those who experience jet lag generally take about one day to recover for each time zone crossed. Older people sometimes require additional time as they are more sensitive to the symptoms of jet lag. Though symptoms will fade without medical intervention, there are behavioral changes and medications that can reduce or possibly prevent the severity of symptoms.

Maintain schedule based on home time zone. If you and your loved one are making a short trip (only one or two days), consider not changing your schedule once you arrive at your destination. Continue to eat and sleep according to your home time zone.

Start shifting sleep time at home. If your trip is longer, you may want to start preparing your loved one for the time change before you leave home. If you are flying west, slowly adjust your sleep schedule so that you are going to bed one to two hours later than usual; if you are flying east, start going to bed one to two hours earlier.

Don't forget sunlight upon arrival. As discussed in Chapter 1, when our eyes see darkness, the pineal gland is signaled to secrete melatonin, which prepares us for sleep. When our eyes sense light, the pineal gland is signaled to stop secreting melatonin, which wakes us up. When you and your loved one arrive at your destination, get into the sunlight as soon as possible. If you arrive at night, expose yourself and your loved one to the early morning sunlight as soon as you both wake up.

Sleep during the flight. It is always better if you can arrive at your destination feeling relatively rested. Consider bringing earplugs, a pillow or a sleep mask for your loved one to allow for a restful night's sleep.

Plan a stopover. If you are traveling across several time zones with your loved one, it may be a good idea to plan a stopover for a couple of days to acclimate to the change in time slowly—again, the more time zones you traverse on your trip, the more severe the symptoms of jet lag and the longer it will take to adjust.

Avoid heavy meals. Eat light meals for the first day or two after arrival. Heavy meals may make your loved one feel drowsy, aggravate gastrointestinal symptoms of jet lag and throw off his or her sleep schedule.

Restrict caffeine use to mornings. Since your loved one's sleep cycle is already disrupted, consuming caffeine should be limited. If he or she can't go without his or her caffeinated beverage of choice, encourage him or her to drink it before lunch so that it doesn't interfere with his or her ability to fall asleep and stay asleep.

Encourage your loved one to take a short nap if necessary. A short nap between 15 and 30 minutes can help restore your loved one's energy and get him or her through the rest of the day. A longer nap is likely to leave your loved one out of sorts and can make it even more difficult for him or her to fall asleep at night.

Consider taking melatonin. The jury is still out on the idea of using melatonin to alleviate jet lag, but a small dose prior to bedtime may decrease your loved one's sleep latency and help him or her stay asleep longer. It's a good idea to talk to your loved one's doctor before incorporating a new supplement into his or her diet. You will want to make sure that melatonin does not counteract or adversely interact with any of your loved one's medications. The doctor can also advise you on suggested dosage. Taking too much melatonin can lead to difficulty waking up and a "mental fog" in the morning.

Try prescription sleep aids. Some travelers who struggle with jet lag find that it helps to take a mild hypnotic (sleeping pill) shortly before bedtime. If your loved one needs extra help falling asleep while traveling, talk to a physician to see if a prescription sleep aid is a good option. Be aware that most doctors do not like to prescribe sleep aids to seniors because they can result in temporary confusion, disorientation and unsteadiness while walking, which all increase the risk of falls.

Before traveling with your older loved one, it's a good idea to take him or her to the doctor for a check-up. The doctor can help ensure that your loved one's health is suitable for travel and that he or she has all the medications that will be needed during the trip.

Jet lag is usually a limited and temporary problem. It occurs only during travel, and it usually resolves on its own. The next chapter will discuss a more enduring sleep problem: snoring. Whether your loved one is the one snoring or the one being kept awake by a snoring companion, he or she is probably not getting the sleep that the body requires. This is an especially important issue to address as snoring can go on indefinitely until you uncover and treat the root cause of the problem. Chapter 7 will examine the reasons why people snore and ways to alleviate the problem. It will also take a look at a condition called obstructive sleep apnea, a potentially life-threatening condition that may develop and worsen as we grow older.

CHAPTER 7: SNORING AND OBSTRUCTIVE SLEEP APNEA

"Laugh and the world laughs with you, snore and you sleep alone."
– *Anthony Burgess*

From the sophisticated wit of authors like Erma Bombeck and Anthony Burgess, to the slapstick comedy of *The Flinstones* and *The Three Stooges*, snoring has certainly found its place in the humor hall of fame. If your loved one can't get a good night's sleep because of snoring, however, he or she may not find it as amusing.

As we grow older, the tissue in the back of our throats loses some of its tone and becomes slack. This can lead to partial or complete airway obstruction, which can in turn lead to snoring or more severely obstructive sleep apnea.

In this chapter, we'll look at what snoring is, the most common causes of snoring and how to find relief. We will also look at a life-threatening condition called obstructive sleep apnea (OSA) —a major symptom of which is snoring—and explain how it is diagnosed and treated.

What Is Snoring?

Snoring is loud breathing during sleep that results from partial or total obstruction of the airway. It is a harsh, rasping, guttural sound that is usually more noticeable when the sleeper inhales, although noise may also occur when the sleeper exhales. Snoring can range from a soft sound that is barely noticeable to a sound loud enough to not only awaken the person snoring, but also the people in other rooms of the house.

It's no surprise then that snoring can often put a strain on intimate relationships. Sometimes, for instance, the partner who doesn't snore chooses to move out of the couple's bedroom in the hopes of getting a better night's sleep. This can leave the partner who snores feeling isolated, angry, helpless and even ashamed and the partner who left feeling lonely and frustrated. Another negative pattern may be created if the non-snorer repeatedly wakes the snorer up during the night to tell him or her, "You're snoring again!" This can be especially frustrating if the person who snores is unaware that he or she does so.

Who Snores?

If you or a loved one snores, you're not alone. Around 50 percent of people over the age of 18 snore at least occasionally and 25 percent are habitual snorers.

Although anyone can develop a problem with snoring, there are certain risk factors that can make the behavior more likely:

- Being male
- Being overweight
- Smoking
- Having a narrow airway
- Drinking alcohol prior to sleep
- Having nasal problems
- Having a family history of snoring
- Growing older

What Causes Snoring?

Snoring can be the result of multiple conditions, some potentially life-threatening and others relatively harmless. Anatomical variations in the structure of the mouth and nose can make some people more prone to snoring. A low, thick palate (the upper part of the mouth) will result in narrower airways and a misaligned jaw can also cause partial obstruction of the airway. Jaw misalignment can either be a natural personal trait, the result of injury or the result of clenching or grinding during sleep (See Chapter 13 about Bruxism). As we age, the tissue in the back of our throats naturally loses its elasticity, which can obstruct the airway. In the nose, if the septum (the thin layer of cartilage that separates the nostrils) is deviated (bent), the likelihood of snoring increases.

You may also notice an increase in snoring if your loved one has a clogged or "stuffy" nose due to an allergy or a cold. Central nervous system depressants, like alcohol, may relax the muscles in the throat, also making snoring more likely.

The most dangerous cause of snoring is obstructive sleep apnea (OSA). This refers to an obstruction of the upper airway severe enough that it actually causes breathing to stop for short periods of time. We will discuss OSA, its diagnosis and its treatment later in this chapter.

Snoring Remedies

If your loved one snores, instruct him or her to try to sleep on his or her side rather than on his or her back. When you sleep on your back, your tongue may drop to the back of your mouth, further obstructing airflow. Encourage your loved one to avoid alcohol and other central nervous system depressants like sedatives and sleeping pills for several hours prior to bedtime. Your loved one may also be interested in checking out over-the-counter products, such as strips that fit over the nose to keep the nostrils open during sleep.

What Are the Risks of Snoring?

A little snoring from time to time probably won't hurt your loved one. Frequent, loud snoring, though, can deprive him or her and you of much-needed sleep. In terms of physical risks, snoring has been correlated with thickening and other abnormalities of the carotid artery. The carotid artery is one of two large blood vessels that supply oxygen and blood to the brain. Narrowing of the carotid artery increases the risk of stroke as well as long-term cognitive decline.

When to See a Doctor about Snoring

Snoring can be much more than a nuisance—as discussed above, it may also have some serious health consequences. If you are providing care to an elderly loved one, listen carefully to how your loved one breathes when he or she is asleep. Soft or occasional snoring is not any cause for alarm, but loud, constant snoring, especially when punctuated with pauses in breathing, warrants a visit to your loved one's doctor. A professional caregiver who stays overnight with your loved one can also check his or her breathing. You should take your loved one to see a doctor to discuss his or her snoring if any of the following conditions exist:

- Your loved one's snoring is often loud enough to awaken or disturb you.
- You have observed pauses in your loved one's breathing during sleep.
- Your loved one wakes up at night choking or gasping for air.
- Your loved one is sleepy during the daytime hours in spite of getting plenty of nighttime sleep (around the recommended 8 hours).
- Your loved one often wakes up in the mornings with headaches or a sore throat.

Obstructive Sleep Apnea (OSA)

OSA is a sleep disorder characterized by frequent pauses in breathing during the night. These pauses are caused by a high concentration of soft tissue around the airway that results from a decrease in muscle tone. When those with OSA breathe during sleep, their airways partially collapse, preventing them from getting the oxygen they need.

The pauses in breathing, called periods of apnea, usually last from ten seconds to a minute or more. A person with OSA may experience as many as five to 30 periods of apnea in a single hour, which could mean 250 periods of apnea in a single night.

Each time apnea occurs, the sleeper awakens briefly to catch his or her breath. Thus, it is practically impossible to get a good night's sleep with untreated OSA.

Diagnosing OSA

Loud snoring and periods of apnea during sleep are usually what bring people with OSA to their doctors. The doctor then performs diagnostic testing. The gold standard for diagnosing OSA is polysomnography, which is administered at a sleep clinic. Your loved one will be hooked up to various pieces of equipment that painlessly monitor the activity of his or her heart, lungs and brain as well as the movements of his or her arms and legs and his or her blood oxygen levels.

There are also home sleep tests available that use less complicated, portable monitoring devices. Home sleep tests are becoming popular because they are less expensive and more convenient than testing in a sleep lab. They do, however, tend to produce false negatives (failing to diagnose OSA when it is actually present). If your loved one's home sleep test is negative but he or she continues to experience symptoms of OSA, the doctor may suggest that your loved one have a full polysomnography at a sleep lab.

OSA Treatments

If your loved one's OSA is not severe, for instance if he or she has only a small number of periods of apnea during the night, your doctor may suggest lifestyle changes such as giving up smoking, maintaining a healthy body weight, exercising regularly and avoiding alcohol and other central nervous system depressants, to ease symptoms.

If your loved one's OSA is more severe, the doctor will probably suggest that he or she use a machine that provides continuous positive airway pressure (CPAP) to keep the airway open during sleep. The positive airway pressure is delivered via a mask that fits over the nose or over the nose and mouth. Some people find the CPAP uncomfortable at first. For example, one patient whose spouse was also receiving CPAP therapy complained that the two of them looked and sounded like "Mr. and Mrs. Darth Vader." A daughter reported that every evening she carefully helped her mother strap on her mask and turn on the CPAP. Every morning when she went into the bedroom to wake her mother up, she found the mask and the machine both neatly placed in the waste paper basket beside the bed.

It may help to try different masks or to experiment with adjusting the straps on the masks to increase comfort. You should also be aware that cognitive decline that can come with age can lead to resistance in using a CPAP or any other unfamiliar equipment. Discourage your loved one from stopping CPAP therapy before speaking to his or her doctor first. Untreated OSA has been correlated with fatigue, diabetes, heart attack and stroke. If your loved one cannot tolerate a CPAP, the doctor may recommend another device like bi-level positive airway pressure (BPAP) or expository positive airway pressure (EPAP). Some people find them to be more comfortable than the CPAP.

If your loved one is resistant, you will probably have to check on him or her frequently during the night. Whenever you find your loved one has removed the mask, replace it gently and offer a simple explanation such as, "Your doctor wants you to wear this all night. It will help you breathe better." While your loved one is getting used to a mechanical device like the CPAP or BPAP, it may be a good idea to hire a caregiver for the nighttime hours so that you do not fall behind on your own sleep.

Surgery may also be used to treat OSA by enlarging the airways in the nose or throat, although most doctors prefer to use this only as a last resort. Some surgical options include repairing a deviated septum in the nose, removing tissue from the back of the throat and repositioning the jaw.

Snoring is a common cause of sleep disturbance, but it is far from the only one. The next chapter will cover a condition called restless legs syndrome, which also impairs sleep quality.

CHAPTER 8: RESTLESS LEGS SYNDROME

"A ruffled mind makes a restless pillow." – *Charlotte Bronte*

Restless legs syndrome (RLS) is a neurobiological condition that causes discomfort in the legs when one is sitting or lying down. The sensations one feels in the calves, thighs and feet are commonly described as creeping, crawling, burning, gnawing and itching. These symptoms are unpleasant and only go away when the afflicted person gets up and moves around.

RLS can begin at any stage of life, including childhood, but symptoms become more pronounced with increasing age. According to the National Institute of Neurological Disorders and Stroke, two to three percent of people over the age of 18 experience moderate to severe RLS symptoms and five percent experience minor symptoms. Women are twice as likely as men to develop RLS.

Causes of RLS

In most cases, the exact cause of RLS is never identified. Though there seems to be a hereditary component, the responsible gene has yet to be isolated. Scientists also suspect hormones may play a role in certain cases because some women experience RLS only during the last trimester of pregnancy. After the baby is born, the RLS symptoms usually disappear within a few weeks. RLS can sometimes be explained by an identifiable condition such as an iron deficiency or advanced kidney failure, though these cases are rare. The good news is that RLS does not shorten one's life expectancy, nor does it herald the onset of a more serious neurological disorder.

RLS Diagnosis

There are no definitive tests that can confirm a diagnosis of RLS. Doctors may, however, order lab work to rule out other conditions. Once this has been done, most doctors feel comfortable diagnosing RLS as long as four criteria are met:

1. The symptoms are most severe at night and improve in the morning.
2. The person feels a strong need to move the affected leg or legs.
3. The disturbing symptoms are triggered by rest, relaxation and attempts to sleep.
4. The sensory symptoms are eased by movement; the relief persists as long as the movement continues.

RLS and Sleep

Because the symptoms of RLS are most intense in the evenings, any effort to lie down and relax is almost impossible. The need to get up and move to alleviate discomfort increases sleep latency. And for up to 80 percent of people with RLS, there is a coexisting disorder called periodic limb movement of sleep (PLMS), which causes twitching, jerking, and kicking of the legs every 15 to 40 seconds throughout the night. If these movements don't awaken the sleeper, they certainly awaken his or her partner.

Interestingly, people who endure horrible RLS symptoms at night usually have a period during the early morning hours when they are essentially symptom-free. This is often one of the only times when people with RLS are able to get some sound sleep, although this early morning nap in no way makes up for a night spent tossing and turning.

Medications Used to Treat RLS

Since there are no medications that have been developed specifically to treat RLS, doctors usually provide medications "off label", which means the medications were developed for other purposes but seem to reduce RLS symptoms. For instance, even though there is no known correlation between Parkinson's disease and RLS, medications developed to ease the symptoms of Parkinson's disease, such as Carbidopa/Levodopa, Mirapex and Requip often relieve the symptoms of RLS as well. Opioids, muscle relaxers, sleeping pills and medications for epilepsy are also used to manage RLS symptoms, but are not encouraged for seniors since they can cause grogginess, confusion, and disrupt balance, all of which can greatly increase the risk of falls.

Most doctors encourage their RLS patients to keep a "symptom diary" to track any medications taken and the dose, daily activities, and severity of symptoms at different times of the day and night. If your loved one is cognitively impaired, you or a caregiver can help him or her keep the diary up-to-date. A frustrating aspect of RLS treatment is that medications that work initially may lose their effectiveness over time. This means that doctors must frequently change doses and medications to maintain symptom control, which is why keeping a journal is important.

Because many people have more than one physician, it's important to tell all of your loved one's doctors about an RLS diagnosis. There are some medications that people with RLS should avoid, such as some classes of antipsychotic medications (haloperidol or phenothiazine-based) and antidepressants that are intended to increase the level of serotonin in the brain. Although the mechanism is not clearly understood, these medications worsen RLS symptoms.

RLS Self Care

Besides medications, there are many home remedies that can sometimes bring relief to people with RLS.

One suggestion is to run a warm or cool bath—depending on your loved one's preferences—before bed and to gently massage his or her legs as he or she sits in the tub. Using warm compresses, cool compresses, or alternating between the two may also ease symptoms.

Some people have found that practicing relaxation techniques like progressive muscle relaxation or meditation is helpful. Others, however, complain that the more they try to relax, the worse the creepy-crawly feelings in their legs become.

Doctors say that a moderate amount of exercise early in the day may help ease symptoms later in the evening. A workout that is too strenuous or too late in the evening, however, may instead make symptoms worse. Your loved one will have to experiment to determine which types of exercise work best for him or her. Some people with RLS find that avoiding caffeine late in the day is helpful. Finally, don't try to keep your loved one from getting out of bed and walking around. When he or she needs to get up and walk or pace for a few minutes, allow him or her to do so.

If your loved one regularly gets up at night and you are not able to be there to monitor him or her, hiring a professional caregiver who can provide supervision and assistance will help give you peace of mind. With help from a caregiver, your loved one can safely move around the house to relieve his or her symptoms and you will be able to sleep soundly knowing that he or she has the full attention of a trained professional.

In the next chapter, we will turn from restless legs to restless minds as we take a look at dreams and nightmares, their causes and various treatments for recurring nightmares and REM sleep behavior disorder.

CHAPTER 9: DREAMS AND NIGHTMARES

"The concept of dreaming is known to the waking mind but to the dreamer there is no waking, no real world, no sanity; there is only the screaming bedlam of sleep." – Akira Kurosawa

Dreams are an involuntary sequence of images, ideas, emotions and sensations that usually occur during REM sleep. They can last anywhere from just a few seconds to 20 minutes or more. Of the eight hours an average person spends sleeping each night, about two are spent dreaming. Researchers estimate that we have between three and five distinct dreams each night.

In spite of all that we do know about dreams, they are still very much a scientific mystery.

Purpose of Dreams

Despite years of research testing multiple hypotheses, scientists are still not sure exactly why we dream, but there are many plausible and fascinating theories.

Sigmund Freud, the father of psychoanalysis, believed that dreams were symbolic clashes between the id, ego and superego, allowing the sleeper to resolve conflicts that were too shocking or emotional to address head-on during normal waking hours.

Other researchers suggest that the brain simply replays images that are retained in long-term memory. We do not always recognize these images because they may occur out of context or as a collage of several different memories that are not connected to each other.

Still another theory is that dreams reinforce and solidify the semantic memories we learn each day. Similarly, others suggest that dreams may be the brain's way of removing repetitive memories and other unnecessary information and developing more efficient neural pathways. As discussed in Chapter 2, sleep seems to play an important role in restorative processes, learning and memory.

Dreams and Memories

Most people remember very few of the details of their dreams. Within five minutes of awakening, the average person can only remember about 50 percent of his or her dreams. Ten minutes after waking up, only about ten percent can be recalled.

Researchers suspect that the rates of forgetfulness are so high because we typically learn through association and repetition. In other words, we remember the things that are connected to other important images and ideas or that we experience frequently. Since dreams are typically vague, disconnected and full of unique images, they are hard to remember.

Nightmares

Nightmares are realistic, disturbing dreams that usually leave the sleeper with feelings of overwhelming fear, anxiety and terror. These emotions may persist, even if the person no longer remembers the specific details of the dream. About two to eight percent of people over the age of 18 have recurring nightmares.

In addition to emotional reactions, nightmares can also cause sleep deprivation, especially if the same nightmare occurs over and over. Severe recurring nightmares are loosely correlated with suicide or attempted self-harm, though cases are rare.

Causes of Nightmares

There are several factors that can increase the occurrence of nightmares.

In a scene from *A Christmas Carol*, Scrooge, upon seeing the ghost of his dead business partner Jacob Marley, scoffs that Jacob is probably a nightmare brought on by a bad meal. "There's more of gravy than grave in you," he quips. Indeed, one cause of nightmares is eating a heavy snack or meal in the evening just before bedtime. As the metabolism works to digest the food, the neurobiological processes in the brain also become more active, eliciting unusual and sometimes frightening images.

Medications that influence brain activity such as narcotics, antidepressants and seizure medications can also produce vivid, bizarre and disturbing dreams.

Physical conditions such as restless legs syndrome and obstructive sleep apnea are also culprits, as are mental conditions such as anxiety, depression and posttraumatic stress disorder. A major life event, such as moving to a new state, or any other unusual amount of stress may also cause nightmares.

Some families tend to have a hereditary tendency towards nightmares, although scientists have not been able to pinpoint a gene.

Treatment of Nightmares

Successful treatment of nightmares depends largely on the
suspected cause. For some, changing the dosage or type of
psychoactive medication they take or working to improve
symptoms of restless legs syndrome, obstructive sleep apnea,
or mental illness can alleviate the problem. For others, imagery
rehearsal is most effective. In this case, the person is asked
to imagine a more positive, less frightening outcome for
the recurring nightmare. For instance, instead of trying to
run from a monster, the dreamer might imagine turning,
confronting it and telling it to go away. This ending gives
the individual a sense of power over frightening dreams.

Dreams and Aging

To date, there has been limited research done on dreams and
nightmares as they relate to seniors and aging. As we mentioned
in Chapter 3, the proportion of REM sleep we experience declines
rapidly after age 70. This decline implies less dreaming, which
means less time to solidify memories and learning, and thus less
time for the brain to do its "housecleaning." However, this may
also mean fewer nightmares, although there are no studies
available to prove this.

If your aging loved one suffers a sudden onset of vivid dreams or
nightmares, it could also be a sign of delirium due to infection,
fever or medication changes. In this instance a trip to the doctor
is warranted for further evaluation.

REM Sleep Behavior Disorder

During normal REM sleep, our muscles are paralyzed so that we do not act out our dreams. Even if we're running towards a friend or family member or being chased by a madman in our dreams, our legs remain stationary in bed. Those with REM sleep behavior disorder, though, physically mimic what they experience in their dreams. This means that they may scream, kick, cry or fight while sleeping.

A recent study conducted at the Mayo Clinic suggests that REM sleep behavior disorder is predictive of the development of neurodegenerative diseases such as Parkinson's disease, Alzheimer's disease and Lewy body disease. However, only about 38 percent of those who experience REM sleep behavior disorder develop a degenerative disease. For those who do, the onset of REM sleep behavior disorder usually occurs at least 15 years prior to the onset of noticeable cognitive decline.

The best treatment for this disorder is a benzodiazepine called clonazepam (Klonopin). Clonazepam is able to reduce or eliminate symptoms in 90 percent of cases. Even though this medication has been effective in eliminating symptoms for the majority of people who suffer from this disorder, there is currently no research as to whether this treatment reverses the decline associated with these neurodegenerative conditions.

The next chapter will look at sleepwalking, which occurs during non-REM (NREM) sleep and is a phenomenon that is correlated with dementia and organic brain syndrome. Topics will include causes of sleepwalking, risks of sleepwalking and suggestions for eliminating sleepwalking.

CHAPTER 10: SLEEPWALKING

"A great perturbation in nature, to receive at once the benefit of sleep, and do the effects of watching!" – *William Shakespeare*

It had been several months since Richard's wife died, but he found he was still having trouble sleeping. He spoke to his doctor, who prescribed zolpidem (Ambien). On the morning after Richard had his first Ambien-induced night's sleep, he woke up to find his kitchen a mess, as if someone had broken into the house in the middle of the night, fixed a meal and left without cleaning up.

The next two nights passed without any problems, but the night after that, Richard awoke sitting in his easy chair. The television was on even though he was sure he had turned it off after the evening news, long before bedtime.

Richard called his doctor to discuss these strange occurrences. His doctor explained that Richard was sleepwalking and that Ambien was the most likely culprit, since he had developed the problem within days of starting the prescription. Due to this unwanted side effect, his doctor discontinued the use of Ambien and prescribed a low dose of Valium, a benzodiazepine, to help Richard sleep better at night. Richard had no further problems with sleepwalking after the medication adjustment.

What Is Sleepwalking?

Sleepwalking, which occurs in about four percent of people over the age of 18, is considered a parasomnia, an undesirable behavior or experience during sleep. Walking is not the only behavior that may occur during sleep. In the example above, Richard actually got up and fixed himself a meal. Other sleepwalkers may try to drive, operate mechanical equipment or engage in other activities that can be quite dangerous in a sleeping state. Aside from getting up and actually walking around the room or the house, sleepwalking behaviors can include:

- Sitting up with a blank look
- Opening eyes during sleep
- Performing any kind of complex task (e.g., driving, fixing a meal, cleaning the bathroom)
- Occasional aggression, especially if startled

Sleepwalking usually occurs early in the night, during the first two cycles of sleep, in the deeper sleep stages (Stage 3 and/or Stage 4). For reasons that are not understood, the brain becomes partially awake, allowing the sleeper to perform complex tasks that he or she normally wouldn't be able to do during these sleep stages. However, the brain is still partially asleep, so sleepwalkers have no awareness of their actions and will not remember them the next morning. The length of a sleepwalking episode can vary from just a few seconds or minutes to more than half an hour. Sleepwalking generally occurs no more than once each night, so if you guide your sleepwalking loved one back to bed, you can be rest assured that he or she will sleep peacefully through the rest of the night. Of course, if your loved one lives alone and does not have someone to walk him or her back to bed, this can be a very dangerous behavior as it can result in a serious fall. If you discover that your loved one is sleepwalking consider hiring an around-the-clock caregiver to come in to ensure he or she is safe throughout the night.

In a recent study of 100 adults who had been diagnosed with sleepwalking, researchers found that 22.8 percent of them sleepwalked on a nightly basis while 43.5 percent sleepwalked at least weekly. The rest sleepwalked sporadically.

What Causes Sleepwalking?

Researchers do not know the exact mechanism that results in sleepwalking. Since it appears to run in families, there may be a genetic component in some cases. In other cases, temporary sleepwalking episodes can be explained by:

- Stressful events
- Strong emotions (positive or negative)
- Sleep deprivation
- Use of alcohol
- Use of certain drugs, including prescription medications
- Intense physical activity in the evening hours

Risks of Sleepwalking

One of the greatest risks of sleepwalking is injury to the sleepwalker. With the brain partially alert and partially in a deep sleep, the sleepwalker has no sense of judgment, especially with regard to safety. He or she may trip and fall while wandering around the house or burn his or her hand while cooking. He or she may also engage in risky behaviors like standing in the middle of the street or driving on the wrong side of the road and disregarding traffic signals.

On rare occasions, sleepwalkers will become aggressive, especially if startled or awakened suddenly. While it is not usually dangerous to wake a sleepwalker, as myths would have you believe, it is best to simply guide your loved one back to bed without waking him or her. If you cannot coax the person to bed, try to awaken your loved one gently and calmly.

In 2013, a research team at the Gui-de-Chauliac Hospital in Montpelier, France compared two groups of 100 adults between the ages of 18 and 58. One group had been diagnosed with sleepwalking; the other group reported no parasomnias. Researchers found that, compared to the group with no parasomnias, the group of people who experienced sleepwalking reported increased daytime sleepiness and fatigue, insomnia, symptoms of depression and anxiety and a perceived poorer quality of life. Prior to these findings, physicians were less apt to take sleepwalking seriously, considering it little more than a nuisance. The French study was the first to show that sleepwalking adults reported mental health issues and a poor quality of life. Doctors are now more likely to acknowledge that sleepwalking is a cause for concern and to prescribe treatments to reduce or eliminate sleepwalking.

Treatments for Sleepwalking

Minimize danger. If you have a loved one who sleepwalks, try to make the home as safe as possible. Make sure your loved one sleeps on the ground floor until the sleepwalking issues are resolved—this could save him or her from a nasty fall down the stairs. Clear away items like electrical cords or loose rugs that could cause tripping and falling in the walkways. Finally, put motion detectors or alarms on all of the doors and windows leading to the outside; if your loved one leaves the house, you'll know about it. If your loved one attempts to drive in his or her sleep, hide the car keys or temporarily disable the car at night. You might also consider hiring a professional caregiver for a few nights to monitor his or her safety.

Talk to your loved one's doctor about medications. The doctor may want to discontinue some medications, such as Ambien, that have been associated with the onset of sleepwalking. The doctor may also want to prescribe medications such as benzodiazepines (Valium) or tricyclic antidepressants (amitriptyline) that have been shown to help reduce or eliminate sleepwalking.

Learn to relax. A counselor, therapist, or other mental health professional can teach your loved one some easy relaxation exercises to do before bed. These exercises can help relieve stress and anxiety, which as mentioned previously can increase the likelihood of sleepwalking episodes. Some sleepwalkers also benefit from being hypnotized and given a post-hypnotic suggestion to remain comfortably in their beds all night.

Try anticipatory awakening. Most sleepwalkers settle into a routine and start sleepwalking at about the same time each night. Identify when your loved one is most likely to get out of bed and start waking him or her up about fifteen minutes before you anticipate the sleepwalking will start. Keep your loved one awake for around 30 to 45 minutes before allowing him or her to resume sleep. This treatment method usually takes one to four weeks before results are noticeable, depending on how long sleepwalking has been occurring and how deeply the pattern is entrenched.

Treat underlying health problems. Sleepwalking can sometimes be related to medical or mental health problems such as restless legs syndrome, posttraumatic stress disorder, partial complex seizures and extreme stress. If a medical or mental health professional is able to treat the underlying issues, the sleepwalking usually also subsides.

Sleepwalking and the Elderly

Some people sleepwalk during childhood and just never stop. Others start sleepwalking in adulthood. Those who begin sleepwalking during their adult years often suffer from more complications with physical health, mood, and behavior than adults who started sleepwalking as children.

Sleepwalking in people over the age of 65 can be an indication of organic brain syndrome, or decreased mental function due to a medical disease. Different types of dementia and associated brain damage can also play a role in sleepwalking. In these cases, the person is usually difficult to arouse and often very confused about where he or she is and what is happening when he or she is awakened. Thus, it is best to gently redirect this person back to bed.

Another health condition that can cause sleepwalking among older adults is an acute infection like a urinary tract infection (UTI) or a high fever. If your loved one's temperature rises, or if he or she starts experiencing nightmares, sleepwalking, or other parasomnias for no apparent reason, make sure your loved one is evaluated by a doctor. A few lab tests and some antibiotics can quickly put an end to the disturbances.

If your loved one regularly sleepwalks or is restless at night, consider hiring a professional caregiver to watch over your loved one while you catch up on some much needed sleep. The caregiver can keep a sleep diary that documents your loved one's nighttime activities, alerting you to any new or disturbing trends in sleeping behavior so that you can visit a doctor. Caregivers also possess the patience and gentleness that is needed to coax your loved one back to bed after a sleepwalking incident.

We mentioned briefly in this chapter how mental health issues like anxiety and depression can both trigger and result from sleepwalking. In the next chapter, we'll take a look at some of the most common mental health issues that can disrupt sleep, how to treat them and how to promote mental health.

CHAPTER 11: MENTAL HEALTH ISSUES

"The best bridge between despair and hope is a good night's sleep."
– E. Joseph Cossman

There are many mental health issues that can interfere with sleep. People with schizophrenia, for instance, might suffer vivid hallucinations and delusions that make them afraid to go to sleep (see Chapter 12 about fear of sleep). People with bipolar disorder who are in the midst of a manic episode might stay awake for several days and nights because they simply don't feel the need to sleep. In this chapter, we'll look closely at three of the most common mental health problems that are deeply entwined with sleep issues: depression, generalized anxiety disorder in the older adult and posttraumatic stress disorder.

Depression

Depression is a word that is misused hundreds of times a day. "I'm so depressed that I have to work on Saturday" or "My team lost the game by three points—how depressing!" In reality, depression is much more than a mild, fleeting case of the blues. To be officially diagnosed with depression, a person must have experienced most of the following symptoms on a daily basis for two weeks or longer:

- Feeling sad or down
- Feeling hopeless
- Losing interest in activities that were once enjoyed
- Withdrawing from friends and family
- Not eating enough or eating too much
- Not sleeping enough or sleeping too much
- Feeling worthless or guilty for no apparent reason
- Thinking about death or suicide

Depression and Insomnia

Insomnia—difficulty falling asleep or waking up too early—is often the symptom that causes people with depression to consult with their doctors. One study conducted in the UK found that 83 percent of depressed patients over the age of 18 experienced insomnia compared to 36 percent of subjects who were not depressed.

In addition to being a symptom, insomnia can also be a precursor of depression. One study followed a group of 7,954 subjects over the age of 18. The researchers interviewed each subject twice with a one-year gap in between. They discovered that 14 percent of subjects who reported insomnia during the first interview had been diagnosed with major depressive disorder by the second interview. Another study, conducted in Michigan, followed 1,200 adults over the age of 18 for three years. The study found that subjects who initially reported insomnia were four times more likely to develop depression over the three-year timespan than those who did not. If symptoms of insomnia persist despite treatment for depression, there is a greater possibility of recurrence than if treatment successfully mitigates all symptoms of depression.

The National Institute of Mental Health (NIMH) reports that 15 percent of seniors over the age of 65 suffer from clinical depression and that 25 percent report being sad on a regular basis. There are a number of life changes that can make seniors susceptible to depression, including retiring from a job that offered a sense of purpose, experiencing the deaths of loved ones, becoming more isolated and feeling an uncomfortable sense of dependence on others because of physical and/or mental impairments. Doctors also suspect that insomnia brought on by illness or injuries may lead to higher rates of depression among seniors.

Be aware that if your loved one is suffering from depression, he or she may be reluctant to talk about it and may avoid using words like "sad" or "depressed". Many seniors are afraid of the stigma that sometimes surrounds mental health issues. Instead of talking about their feelings, depressed seniors may complain about physical aches and pains such as arthritis, headaches or muscle aches. Other symptoms of depression specific to the senior population include anxiety, memory problems, slow movements and speech, irritability and neglecting personal care.

If you suspect your loved one is depressed, try to convince him or her to talk to a doctor or mental health professional. If your loved one lives alone, consider hiring a caregiver to provide social stimulation, emotional support and companionship. Because so many depressed seniors suffer from insomnia, it may also be a good idea to have a caregiver present at night to soothe your loved one when he or she can't sleep.

Depression and Hypersomnia

About 10 to 20 percent of people with depression experience a condition called hypersomnia, defined as excessive daytime sleepiness over a period of at least three months. Those with hypersomnia may sleep through their alarm clocks and be late to work on a regular basis, or they may require one or more naps during the day in order to be able to function. Hypersomnia is considered a feature of atypical depression. People with atypical depression also tend to overeat and complain that their arms and legs feel heavy. Because they often spend a great deal of time in bed, they may have trouble maintaining relationships. Atypical depression is far more prevalent among those under the age of 30 than older adults. The treatments are the same for people with any other kind of depression: medication, therapy and lifestyle changes.

Sleep Deprivation and Relief of Depression Symptoms

A few years ago, scientists made an interesting discovery: when they prevented people with depression from falling asleep, about 60 to 70 percent experienced a measurable improvement in mood; some even achieved a complete remission of symptoms. Unfortunately, the improved mood lasted only as long as the subjects could be kept awake and given the negative health outcomes associated with sleep deprivation (see Chapter 2), the method was impractical as a long-term treatment. Researchers have, however, continued to study the phenomenon in the hopes of developing new treatments for depression.

Treating Insomnia Caused by Depression

If your loved one is experiencing insomnia as a symptom of depression there are a number of potential lifestyle changes that he or she can make. People with depression tend to do better with a closely regulated sleep schedule so going to bed and awakening at a consistent time is helpful. It's also a good idea to spend some time outdoors in the sunlight. This can help reset the biological sleep clock and get your loved one back into a normal circadian rhythm. Moderate exercise in the morning or afternoon may be helpful, but vigorous exercise late in the day may cause over-arousal and make your loved one's sleep problems even worse. Try steering your loved one away from watching television in the evening. Many of the programs are suspenseful, violent, or otherwise over-stimulating and may keep him or her awake. If your loved one can't sleep, encourage him or her to get out of bed. Suggest a relaxing activity like reading a book, working on a crossword puzzle, or taking a warm bath. When your loved one feels tired, you can help him or her go back to bed. Finally, save the bedroom for sleep. You don't want your loved one's bedroom associated with reading, watching TV, working, or any other wakeful activity.

Generalized Anxiety Disorder (GAD)

Laura was 16 when she married her high school sweetheart, Jerry. Shy and unassuming, she always counted on Jerry to lead the household, take care of finances and make the majority of decisions for the family. The system worked well until Jerry passed away from a stroke at the age of 83.

Both of their adult sons lived out of town and Laura didn't want to burden them with her problems, but she felt completely lost without Jerry. She hesitated to make financial decisions for fear she would make a terrible error that would cost her the retirement money she and Jerry had so carefully saved.

When she tried to sleep at night, her mind raced with all the things that could possibly go wrong with the house. She often lay awake until morning worrying.

Soon she became frightened of making almost any decision at all. Even a simple choice like going to play Bingo with friends or staying home was so anxiety-provoking that it nearly brought her to tears.

When she visited her doctor, Laura was diagnosed with generalized anxiety disorder. Researchers believe that 10 to 20 percent of the population over the age of 60 has some form of anxiety disorder. Among people over the age of 18, anxiety is the most common type of mental health issue for women and the second most common type (after alcohol and drug abuse) for men.

The symptoms of GAD include persistent worrying, often without a legitimate cause, trouble relaxing, problems falling asleep and staying asleep and difficulty concentrating. People with GAD also often have an exaggerated startle reflex. Older adults are more likely than younger adults to experience physical anxiety symptoms such as chest pains and headaches.

What Causes GAD?

Laura's GAD was brought on or exacerbated by the trauma and grief of her husband's death. Other causes may include:

- Caffeine
- Alcohol or drugs
- Family history of anxiety
- Neurodegenerative disease (e.g., Alzheimer's disease)
- Other physical or mental illnesses

Sometimes, fears about the aging process itself can result in GAD. Older adults may be concerned about falling or becoming ill and not being able to call for help, taking sole responsibility of paying for medical care or for their mortgages or the possibility of ending up alone in a nursing home.

Treating GAD

The best treatment for GAD in seniors is a combination of medication, therapy and social support. Medication will not cure GAD, but it will control the symptoms while your loved one learns new coping skills in therapy. Benzodiazepines work quickly, but they can also make your loved one feel confused and unsteady on his or her feet. To avoid these side effects, many doctors prefer to prescribe a type of antidepressant called a selective serotonin reuptake inhibitor (SSRI) such as Prozac.

Counseling can help your loved one learn different relaxation techniques and productive ways of addressing worries. Social support is another vital component of treatment. If your senior loved one has few friends or family members close by, consider hiring a caregiver who can visit with your loved one, plan outings and help keep your loved one engaged in the community.

Posttraumatic Stress Disorder (PTSD)

Posttraumatic stress disorder is a condition that some people experience after living through or witnessing a trauma such as a battle, an attack, or a natural or human-made disaster. Although not everyone who experiences a traumatic event develops PTSD, many do. Some people continue to experience PTSD symptoms long after the trauma has occurred. Many Vietnam veterans, for instance, still meet diagnostic criteria for PTSD more than 40 years after their experiences in combat. Other people start experiencing PTSD symptoms for the first time many years after the original trauma has occurred.

Factors of late-onset PTSD include:

- **Retirement.** Not working gives people more time to dwell on emotional upsets.

- **Declines in health.** Health problems can lead trauma survivors to feel weaker and less capable of protecting themselves and their loved ones.

- **Television news.** By showing scenes of war and other types of violence, television can trigger old memories.

- **Stopping alcohol or illicit drug use.** If your loved one has been using alcohol or other drugs to deal with the trauma, cutting back or stopping these substances can allow PTSD symptoms to surface.

Some of the symptoms of PTSD include flashbacks, nightmares about the trauma, hyper-vigilance and avoidance of people, places and situations reminiscent of the trauma. For instance, Hal and his twin brother Alan served together in Vietnam. Although the brothers had been very close growing up, after the war they could never stand to spend much time with one another. Seeing each other brought back too many unpleasant memories of the war. Sleep disturbance is an especially common symptom of PTSD. In fact one study found that 92.5 percent of soldiers diagnosed with PTSD reported sleep problems.

Sleep Issues and PTSD

PTSD can interfere with sleep in a variety of ways. Falling asleep can be very difficult because of hyper-arousal or hyper-vigilance. If the trauma resulted in painful injuries, these, too, can prevent sleep. People with PTSD may also have trouble staying asleep. They frequently experience intense nightmares about the trauma that awaken them in the middle of the night. Other people with PTSD lose their ability to reach deep sleep (Stage 3 and Stage 4). This means that they are often easily awoken during the night. Finally, PTSD often co-occurs with other sleep disorders such as restless legs syndrome and obstructive sleep apnea.

Treating PTSD

One of the first steps in the successful treatment of PTSD is ensuring that any other co-existing medical problems are treated. Next, doctors may prescribe medications like benzodiazepines or antidepressants to alleviate PTSD symptoms. Finally, people with PTSD are encouraged to talk about their traumatic experiences with a therapist or a support group. Some people with PTSD find that keeping a journal is therapeutic and provides them with a safe place to record their feelings about the trauma and its aftermath.

Some of the suggestions that ease insomnia with depression are also effective in fighting insomnia with PTSD. These include:

- Moderate exercise in the morning or afternoon
- Time spent outdoors in sunlight
- Avoidance of alcohol, caffeine and nicotine prior to bedtime

PTSD and Dementia

A longitudinal study published in the *Archives of General Psychiatry* suggests that PTSD may predict the onset of dementia. The study examined the medical records of 181,093 veterans over the age of 55 spanning seven years. Researchers determined that those with PTSD ran a 10.6 percent risk of developing dementia while those without PTSD ran a 6.6 percent risk. These figures remained the same even after controlling for issues like head trauma and drug and alcohol addiction. Researchers are now trying to determine if successfully treating PTSD early in life can reduce the risk for developing dementia.

Most of the people described in the previous chapters want to sleep but find themselves unable to do so. The next chapter will look at people who, for the most part, want to stay awake. These people are victims of hypnophobia, or an irrational fear of falling asleep.

CHAPTER 12: FEAR OF SLEEP

"I never sleep cause sleep is the cousin of death." – *Nasir Jones*

Seventy-two-year-old Ben had always managed to get a restful night's sleep until the morning he awoke to find that his beloved wife, Sandra, had passed away beside him during the night.

After that, Ben began to dread bedtime. He often lay awake wondering if there was any way he could have saved Sandra if he had woken up earlier. He began to wonder what else he might miss during his restful slumbers. When he did sleep, he was tormented with nightmares about finding Sandra dead. Eventually just sitting in bed became anxiety-provoking.

Ben was fast developing a case of hypnophobia, or fear of sleep. People with hypnophobia do whatever they can to delay or avoid falling asleep. They may use caffeine or other drugs to keep themselves awake. The resulting sleep deprivation only worsens their anxiety and mental anguish.

There have not been any formal studies done to assess how many people suffer from hypnophobia, but primary care physicians say that it is a complaint they hear about regularly.

Causes of Fear of Sleep

There are many reasons why people may come to fear bedtime and falling asleep. One of the most commonly cited reasons is recurring nightmares. Some people, like Ben, dream about tragic events that actually happened. Other people have recurring bad dreams about events that have not actually occurred but that they fear, such as falling from a great height or being chased. Real or not, the dreams are horrifying enough to make those who experience them want to avoid sleep.

Another reason for hypnophobia is a fear of the lack of control that occurs while sleeping. Thoughts may center on potential intruders having the upper hand while the person sleeps defenselessly. Some of these people may have actually experienced the terror of being attacked while asleep. Others may know someone who was victimized during sleep, or they might have read about such attacks or seen segments about them on television.

Along a similar vein, hypnophobia can result from actually having slept through a traumatic event as Ben did. Sixty-one-year-old Barbara, for instance, went to sleep around 9:00 PM on Wednesday as she always did. She slept peacefully through the night, but when she woke up on Thursday morning, she found her home had been burglarized while she slept. The thought that she could sleep through something like that—and the fear of what might have happened had she arisen during the burglary—haunted Barbara and made it difficult for her to fall asleep. She kept imagining she heard her door being opened or footsteps in the hallway.

In certain cases, those who fear sleep have suffered a traumatic event that had nothing to do with sleep or bedtime. However, when they lie down at night and try to relax, memories of the trauma come flooding back. Soon these people come to associate sleepiness with their horrible memories.

Finally, some people are afraid that they might die in their sleep. This fear can affect anyone, but it is often especially strong in people with serious health conditions such as heart or lung disease or obstructive sleep apnea.

Treatments for Hypnophobia

The treatment for fear of sleep depends very much on the circumstances under which the fear developed. That said, it's a good idea for treatment to start with a visit to your loved one's doctor to rule out any underlying medical issues that may contribute to the fear. Someone who is afraid to sleep because he or she wakes up coughing and gagging, for instance, might have a condition like obstructive sleep apnea that can easily be treated. The doctor may also prescribe benzodiazepines and/or antidepressants to control symptoms quickly before suggesting interventions like talk therapy or better sleep hygiene.

One type of therapy that is particularly helpful in treating hypnophobia is cognitive behavioral therapy (CBT). Cognitive behavioral therapy encourages people to examine beliefs about certain life events and determine if the beliefs are realistic. For instance, someone like Ben might be encouraged to seek out the facts about his wife's death and whether—realistically—he could have saved her. Cognitive behavioral therapy requires that the client be able to understand and process new information. Thus, it is not usually a good treatment choice for someone who suffers from Alzheimer's or other forms of dementia.

Support groups are another great therapeutic platform for those with hypnophobia. They are especially helpful for people who have been through traumatic events, offering emotional support and reducing feelings of isolation. Also, talking about the trauma one has endured may help discharge emotions and fears so that they do not build up and interfere with the ability to relax and rest.

People who tend to lie awake and worry about bad things that might happen while they sleep often respond well to relaxation training such as progressive muscle relaxation (PMR) and transcendental meditation. Learning to relax can help banish negative thoughts and help sleep come more easily. Others find comfort in taking concrete steps to address and alleviate their fears. Someone who is afraid of becoming ill or injured at night and not being able to call for help, for instance, might decide to purchase a personal medical alarm that he or she can use to summon help from anywhere in the home. Barbara, whose home was burglarized while she slept, adopted a two-year-old boxer from the local animal shelter. She was able to rest more easily knowing her dog would alert her if someone attempted to break in again.

Those who struggle with nightmares, especially those who have the same bad dream over and over, might benefit from imagery rehearsal. Discussed in more detail in Chapter 9, imagery rehearsal is a way to gain control over nightmares by visualizing different, more positive outcomes to bad dreams.

Finally, some people sleep more comfortably with another person in the house. If your senior loved one lives alone, you might want to consider hiring a caregiver to stay with him or her through the night. The caregiver can provide companionship, support and practical assistance, which would help ease the individual's fears.

There is no specific research on older adults and hypnophobia. There is, however, anecdotal evidence to suggest that seniors have less fear of dying in their sleep than do younger people.

This chapter looked at the difficulties experienced by people who fear sleep for a variety of reasons. The next chapter examines another disorder that makes quality sleep challenging called bruxism. Bruxism causes people to clench or grind their teeth at night. Not only is it hard on the teeth and the jaw, but it can also cause insomnia and other changes in sleep patterns.

CHAPTER 13: BRUXISM

"Not being able to sleep is terrible. You have all the misery of having partied all night...without the satisfaction." – *Lynn Johnston*

Sleep bruxism is a movement disorder that causes people to grind their teeth together and/or clench their jaws while sleeping. The disorder is mainly present in children under the age of 18. Within this age group, the condition usually resolves on its own during adolescence without the need for treatment. Some children, however, continue to experience episodes of sleep bruxism into their adult years. In other cases, adults spontaneously develop sleep bruxism; studies suggest that between eight and ten percent of adults over the age of 18 deal with sleep bruxism on a regular basis.

Causes of Sleep Bruxism

The causes of sleep bruxism have not been confirmed, but researchers have several educated guesses including stress, anger, or other negative mental states or having an abnormal bite that prevents proper alignment of the upper and lower teeth. Neurodegenerative disorders, such as Huntington's disease or Parkinson's disease, have also been associated with bruxism. Teeth grinding may also be a rare side effect of some psychiatric medications including older antipsychotics and antidepressants. If your loved one has been diagnosed with a neurodegenerative disorder like Parkinson's disease, you may want to proactively inquire about the possibility of bruxism, prevention and/or treatment. Also consult your loved one's physician and pharmacist about whether teeth grinding may be a side effect of any prescribed medications or their interactions.

How Is Sleep Bruxism Diagnosed?

For many adults, the first indication they are clenching their jaws or gnashing their teeth at night comes from their significant other; enamel on enamel makes an unpleasant grinding sound that can keep a partner awake at night. For those who live alone, the first noticeable symptoms may be increased tooth sensitivity and tenderness or soreness in jaw muscles. Sleep bruxism can also cause earaches and headaches. In all cases, a dental exam will usually reveal heavy wear and tear on the teeth, including flattened, broken, or chipped surfaces.

Once sleep bruxism is suspected, the next step is usually participation in an overnight sleep study in a lab. This is done because bruxism has been linked to disorders like obstructive sleep apnea and restless legs syndrome and your loved one's doctor will want to make sure that all sleep-related problems are properly identified and treated.

Treating Sleep Bruxism

Many treatments for sleep bruxism have been proposed over the years, but not all have been successful. The British website **Bruxism.org.uk** provides a literature review of the most effective interventions, which include:

Occlusal splints. Also known as bite guards, bruxism appliances and bite plates, occlusal splints are removable dental devices that cover the teeth and gums to prevent damage and stabilize the jaw. Bruxism.org.uk considers occlusal splints the treatment of choice for sleep bruxism because they are carefully molded to fit the wearer's teeth and protect them from further wear. Occlusal splints, however, do not cure bruxism; they only seek to minimize the harm caused by the condition.

Hypnosis. Hypnosis involves coaching people into a deeply relaxed and suggestible state. Once the patient is in this state, the hypnotist makes one or more post-hypnotic suggestions, like encouraging a patient to open and close his or her hand when stressed instead of grinding his or her teeth. Research suggests that this technique is not always successful, but the people who do benefit report almost total relief of symptoms. The effects seem to be long-term, lasting up to three years after the final hypnotic treatment.

Mandibular advancement devices (MADs). The mandibular advancement device was designed primarily to treat snoring and obstructive sleep apnea. It is a mouthpiece that holds the tongue and the lower jaw forward in order to open up additional space in the throat cavity, enabling those wearing the device to breathe more easily. Research suggests that using a MAD can result in a significant reduction of chewing and grinding behaviors at night. Unfortunately, two-thirds of subjects reported finding MADs painful to wear. This discomfort may have inhibited bruxism activity, but it makes MADs less than ideal as a treatment option.

Muscle relaxers. Also known as muscle relaxants, these medications can temporarily ease tension in the jaw and prevent bruxism symptoms. Long-term use is not recommended, however, due to the number of side effects and the risk of addiction to the medication. In one study, for instance, two-thirds of the subjects taking muscle relaxers stopped use because they found the side effects such as drowsiness, dry mouth and urinary retention intolerable.

Sleep hygiene. Improving sleep hygiene through tactics such as avoiding stimulants before bedtime and maintaining a regular sleep schedule is an intuitively appealing solution. In theory, these practices lead to better sleep, which means that more sleep time is spent in deep sleep (Stage 3 and Stage 4). This would likely reduce bruxism, which occurs mainly in the earlier sleep stages. There have not been any formal studies assessing the effectiveness of sleep hygiene as an intervention to reduce bruxism, however, so for now it is not a verified treatment.

Over the last section of this book, we've looked at many barriers to sleep including occasional insomnia, snoring, obstructive sleep apnea, sleepwalking, restless legs syndrome, mental health issues and sleep bruxism.

In the next section, we're going to turn our attention away from sleep disorders and look instead at healthy sleep habits. We'll provide tips for eating a sleep-healthy diet, suggest 25 ways to relax, 12 activities to avoid before bedtime and discuss medications and holistic remedies that may help improve the quality of sleep.

CHAPTER 14: ADOPTING A SLEEP-HEALTHY DIET

"To sup well is to live well, and that's the way to sleep well."
– Sir Thomas Overbury

Home Care Assistance, the leading provider of in-home care, uses a proprietary, holistic approach to care and aging called the Balanced Care Method™ (BCM). The BCM is based on scientific studies of the long-living, healthy elders in the Okinawa region of Japan. A key component of healthy longevity in this region is diet. As a result, all Home Care Assistance caregivers receive culinary training through the company's online university to create healthy and delicious meals for their clients that contain vegetables, whole grains, lean proteins, flavonoids and omega-3 fatty acids. These foods are easy to digest and help clients achieve a restful night's sleep. You, too, can help prepare your loved one for sleep by following the suggestions below.

Simple Rules for Bedtime Eating and Drinking

Eating certain types of food at bedtime can make a big difference —positive or negative—in your loved one's quality of sleep that night. For the best sleep possible, suggest the following:

1. **Make sure your loved one isn't hungry.** Ensure your loved one feels full and satisfied at bedtime. Otherwise, he or she will have a hard time falling asleep and may wake up early due to hunger pangs.

2. **Offer a light snack.** The ideal choice will contain carbohydrates, proteins and tryptophan (an essential amino acid found in foods like egg whites and turkey), as these compounds will signal the body that it is time to prepare for sleep. In the body, tryptophan converts to serotonin and, from that, to melatonin. See the next section for some specific ideas.

3. **Make sure your loved one doesn't drink too many fluids before bedtime.** Your loved one's sleep cycle will be disrupted every time he or she has to get up at night to use the bathroom. In addition, getting out of bed and going to the bathroom in darkness poses a fall risk.

4. **Avoid large, high-fat meals late in the day.** They can cause unpleasant dreams that may wake your loved one up at night. If your loved one needs assistance in preparing well-balanced meals that are low in fat, consider hiring a caregiver. Home Care Assistance caregivers are trained in healthy meal preparation and our *Comfort Foods Cookbook* contains a multitude of delicious, nutritious recipes that appeal to all palates.

5. **Steer clear of nicotine and caffeine before bedtime.** These are both stimulants and can increase sleep latency.

6. **Avoid alcohol before bedtime.** While alcohol may help one fall asleep more quickly, it is likely to make your loved one restless and wakeful later at night, disrupting the quality and duration of sleep.

Foods That Enhance Sleep

If your loved one is craving a bedtime snack, try one of these foods:

Fish. Fish like salmon, halibut and tuna all contain vitamin B6, which the body needs to make melatonin, the "sleep hormone."

Kale. Kale and other green, leafy vegetables are also important sources of vitamin B6.

Yogurt. Yogurt and other nonfat dairy products are packed with calcium. A calcium deficiency can make it harder to fall asleep. If your loved one has trouble falling asleep, consider giving him or her a glass of milk, served warm or cold, before bedtime.

Whole grains. Whole grains contain a healthy amount of magnesium. A magnesium deficiency makes it harder to maintain sleep and to reach the deeper levels of sleep. Consider giving your loved one a magnesium supplement, which can be purchased at many grocery and health food stores. Be sure to consult with his or her physician first before making any changes to your loved one's diet.

Almonds. Almonds are high in magnesium, and they contain protein to help maintain a steady blood glucose (sugar) level throughout the night.

Chamomile tea or decaffeinated green tea. If your loved one enjoys a warm drink before bed, try herbal or decaffeinated teas. Chamomile tea is soothing and can induce sleep quickly. Green tea contains theanine, which decreases sleep latency. If your loved one does drink tea, remember to limit intake to one cup. You don't want to counteract the positive effects of the teas with frequent bathroom breaks throughout the night.

Bananas. Bananas are rich in potassium, which can help relax tight, stressed muscles. Bananas also contain magnesium and are high in tryptophan.

Oatmeal. Oatmeal is a good, old-fashioned comfort food. It is warm, relaxing, easy to prepare and light on the stomach. It also contains calcium, magnesium and potassium. If your loved one does eat oatmeal in the evening, go light on sweeteners like maple syrup or agave nectar.

Hard-boiled egg. A protein-rich egg will help control blood glucose levels throughout the night.

Cherries. Cherries are one of the only natural food sources of melatonin. Unfortunately, they are only in season for about two months during the summer. If you don't happen to catch that lucky two-month window, a cup of tart cherry juice one hour before bedtime can produce the same sleep-inducing effect.

Warm milk. Dieticians have been going back and forth for years about whether this is a real sleep food or simply an old wives' tale. The bottom line is that it probably doesn't have all the magical powers people suggest, but it is a comfort food that is high in calcium and contains tryptophan. Again, remember to limit intake so as not to increase the need for urination throughout the night.

Dates. Dates are the perfect marriage between tryptophan and carbohydrates—tryptophan tends to be absorbed best with carbohydrates.

Cottage cheese. Cottage cheese is a slowly digested protein that helps keep the digestive system relaxed during sleep. It also contains tryptophan. Eating about a half-cup of cottage cheese in the evening should give your loved one several hours of comfortable sleep.

Peanuts and peanut butter. Both peanuts and peanut butter are good sources of protein. They are also packed with niacin, which promotes the release of serotonin in the brain. Lack of serotonin has been implicated in both depression and sleep problems.

Grapes. Like cherries, grapes also contain melatonin. Regular ingestion will encourage a regular sleep-wake cycle. Grapes are also a great food to take on trips as they help ease the effects of jet lag.

Scallops. Scallops are full of tryptophan, magnesium and vitamin B3. Vitamin B3, also known as niacin, can help your loved one relax and get ready for sleep.

Pumpkin seeds. Pumpkin seeds are high in magnesium. Although researchers are not sure why, pumpkin seeds also seem to have the ability to calm the body.

Chickpeas. Chickpeas are high in protein. They also give a little boost to serotonin as well as to vitamin B6.

Honey. A teaspoonful of honey can raise blood sugar just enough to reduce the production of orexin, a neurotransmitter that promotes wakefulness.

Dark chocolate. Eating dark chocolate reduces production of cortisol, an inflammatory chemical in the brain also known as the "stress hormone". Though this effect promotes calm, the caffeine in dark chocolate can inhibit sleep. Thus, limit ingestion to daytime hours and not right before bedtime.

Edamame. Just one cup of edamame has 122 percent of the daily recommended values of tryptophan.

Kiwi. Kiwi is a tasty fruit whose high levels of antioxidants can help the body get rid of free radicals that may disrupt the regular sleep cycle. They are also packed with serotonin, which improves mood and supports better sleep.

Flax seeds. Flax seeds have high levels of tryptophan and magnesium. They are also a great source of omega-3 fatty acids, which can reduce symptoms of anxiety, depression and stress.

Non-fat popcorn. Non-fat popcorn is a carbohydrate, which helps bring tryptophan to the brain. For best results, combine popcorn with a tryptophan- or protein-rich food such as warm milk or peanut butter.

Vanilla ice cream. For those with a sweet tooth, a small dish of vanilla ice cream contains tryptophan, calcium, protein and carbohydrates. Top with slivered almonds to get even more nutrients. Remember to avoid chocolate ice cream in the evening hours as it contains caffeine.

There are many foods and combinations of foods that can help ensure a good night's rest.

Sometimes dietary changes, however, aren't enough to do the trick by themselves. The next chapter looks at medications that are often prescribed or purchased over-the-counter to help with sleep.

CHAPTER 15: SEDATIVES AND HYPNOTICS

"Also, I could finally sleep. And this was the real gift, because when you cannot sleep, you cannot get yourself out of the ditch—there's not a chance." – Elizabeth Gilbert

Throughout this book, we've mentioned that there are times when your doctor might consider prescribing medication to help your loved one go to sleep and stay asleep. This chapter takes a look at the different medications that are available to help with sleep and their effects on the elderly, if known.

Please do not use this chapter as a substitute for the advice of a physician or other medical professional. Nothing can replace the recommendation of an expert physician who is familiar with your loved one's background and care. Rather, think of this chapter as a reference or as a way to start a conversation with your loved one and his or her physician.

Many older adults use medication to treat insomnia. In 2011, for instance, 60 million prescriptions were written for sleep aids. Forty million of those prescriptions were for products with zolpidem, more popularly known as Ambien. Since Ambien is one of the most commonly prescribed sleep aids, we will address this product first.

Ambien (zolpidem)

As a leading prescribed sleep aid, Ambien first became popular for its ability to reduce sleep latency. Unfortunately, its effects did not last long enough to sustain sleep throughout the night, and people taking it began to report bizarre behaviors like sleepwalking and attempting other complex tasks in their sleep (see Chapter 10). The manufacturers soon came out with Ambien CR (continued release), which was intended to help users fall asleep and stay asleep throughout the night. Although Ambien is generally considered safe, between 2005 and 2010, ER visits related to its use increased 220 percent. The most frequently cited complaints were increased drowsiness or interaction with other drugs. In 2013, the FDA required that Ambien doses for women be cut in half to avoid next day sleepiness.

Lunesta (eszopiclone)

Lunesta is a short-acting sedative that works by slowing brain activity to allow for relaxation and sleep. It works on most people within 30 minutes; some people claim to have fallen asleep only 15 to 20 minutes after taking it. Its manufacturers claim that it is safe for short-term use in the elderly.

Rozerem (ramelteon)

A melatonin-receptor agonist, Rozerem functions much like melatonin in the brain. It has been approved by the FDA for long-term use, and carries no risk of dependence, withdrawal symptoms, or rebound insomnia (insomnia that gets worse after one stops taking medication). Studies show that it can reduce sleep latency by 15 to 20 minutes. Unfortunately, the benefits do not last. After four weeks, people who take Rozerem sleep no longer than those who take a placebo for four weeks.

Sinequan (doxepin)

Sinequan is an older medication used to treat both depression and anxiety disorders. The FDA has also approved use in small doses—3mg to 6mg—to treat insomnia.

Benzodiazepines

Some of the more popular benzodiazepines include Xanax, Valium and Ativan. They are used as sedatives to help calm people who are anxious and as hypnotics to help induce sleep. Side effects include cognitive impairments, lingering drowsiness and unsteadiness. They have been known to increase the risk of falls and hip fractures among elderly patients. Therefore, they are generally not recommended for seniors, especially those with cognitive impairments.

Tricyclic Antidepressants

Tricyclic antidepressants are an older class of antidepressants with sedative properties. Some of the more popular choices today include Amitriptyline, Imipramine and Trazadone. Side effects may include drowsiness, constipation and dry mouth. Because small doses of tricyclic antidepressants can effectively treat insomnia, most people do not experience severe side effects.

Over-the-Counter Medications

Some sleep aids such as Unisom are available over-the-counter. These sleep aids typically contain antihistamines which cause drowsiness and reduce sleep latency. They are recommended only for short-term use. Because side effects include drowsiness that lasts into the next day, they are generally not recommended for elderly adults.

The past two chapters have looked at different foods that may help your loved one get a better night's sleep and medications that are frequently prescribed to decrease sleep latency and maintain sleep through the night. The next chapter will examine some alternative remedies for insomnia and other sleep problems.

CHAPTER 16: ALTERNATIVE REMEDIES

"Turn resolutely to work, to recreation, or in any case to physical exercise till you are so tired you can't help going to sleep and when you wake up, you won't want to worry." – B.C. Forbes

Over the course of this book, we've introduced a number of holistic remedies that can help people fall and stay asleep. Examples include taking a warm bath prior to bedtime, using aromatherapy and practicing progressive muscle relaxation.

In this chapter, we'll look at alternative medications that work with the body to decrease sleep latency and improve the quality of sleep. Most of them are available over-the-counter and can be found in health food stores. Of course it is always important to talk to your loved one's physician and pharmacist before introducing these options to avoid potential negative side effects and medication interactions. Make sure the doctor has a complete list of all of your loved one's current medicines, including eye drops, nose drops, vitamins and herbal supplements. Although alternative remedies are usually quite safe, they are potent and can interact with other medications your loved one is taking. For instance, if your loved one is taking antidepressants to increase serotonin levels and then starts taking a new medication that also increases serotonin levels, he or she may develop too much serotonin in the body, a potentially fatal condition called serotonin syndrome.

5-HTP

5-HTP is a pill containing tryptophan, which helps the body manufacture serotonin, a neurotransmitter. Unlike serotonin supplements, 5-HTP is able to cross from the bloodstream into the brain. Thus, it has the effect of actually raising serotonin levels inside the brain. The standard dosage of 5-HTP is 100mg per night. 5-HTP appears to work best for people whose insomnia is related to depression.

Melatonin

As we mentioned in Chapter 1, melatonin is released in the brain in response to darkness and helps relax the body in preparation for sleep. As people age, they produce less melatonin. Scientists believe this is one reason why older adults don't sleep as well as young adults. Melatonin is available as a supplement. The recommended dosage is 1mg to 3mg taken 90 minutes to two hours before bedtime.

Valerian root

Valerian contains chemicals called valepotriates that act as strong muscle relaxers and sedatives. Taking valerian increases the time spent in deep sleep and REM sleep, which naturally decreases as we age. There is no gold standard as far as dosages go, but most studies assessing its effectiveness used between 400mg and 900mg.

Passion flower

If your loved one suffers from insomnia caused by worry, over-work and over-exhaustion, passion flower tea may help. Offer your loved one three glasses of the tea throughout the day, with the last serving about an hour before bedtime; monitor your loved one over a period of a few days and see if the insomnia symptoms improve.

Theanine

Theanine is an amino acid found in green tea. It does not sedate, but it calms the mind and improves mood and cognition. One Japanese study found that subjects given 200mg of theanine at bedtime spent more time in quality sleep than subjects given placebos.

California poppy

California poppy helps people who are restless and anxious fall asleep and improves the quality of their sleep. It can be taken with valerian or taken alone as a tincture of 30 to 40 drops daily.

Hops

Hops is a fast-acting sedative that is used for anxiety, panic attacks and other stress-related conditions. It can be taken as a tincture or a tea (Note: because hops contains steroids, discussing usage with your loved one's physician and pharmacist is especially important).

Magnolia bark

Magnolia bark is used to treat morning insomnia (waking up too early and being unable to fall back to sleep). Magnolia bark works by decreasing cortisol levels in the body. (Cortisol has an excitatory function and prepares the body to get up and move in the morning.) It is generally taken as a 200mg tablet or capsule taken before bedtime.

Ashwagandha

Ashwagandha treats stress and delays the release of cortisol in the morning. The typical dosage is 500mg per day.

Keep a close eye on your loved one for the first several days after he or she starts taking one or more of the aforementioned alternative medications. Look for potential warning signs like increased confusion, gastrointestinal problems (nausea, vomiting, diarrhea), getting too much sleep or not sleeping at all. If your loved one shows any of these signs, consult with a doctor immediately.

The next step in ensuring your loved one gets restful sleep is developing a relaxation routine or list of activities to do just before it is time to go to sleep. The more soothing evening activities you can tap into, the greater your chances of finding one or more that calms your loved one and gets him or her ready for a nice, long night of sleep.

Chapter 17 examines 25 ways to relax before bedtime. Of course not all of these methods will work for every single person—we wouldn't expect them to—but if you can use this list to identify half a dozen relaxation techniques that are especially helpful for your loved one, you'll be well on your way to re-establishing a normal sleep cycle for him or her.

CHAPTER 17: 25 WAYS TO RELAX BEFORE BEDTIME

"Finish each day before you begin the next, and interpose a solid wall of sleep between the two." – Ralph Waldo Emerson

At several different times in this book, we've talked about the importance of good sleep hygiene. In this chapter, we'll examine a variety of methods so that you and your loved one can find what works best. Look over this list of 25 suggestions that may reduce sleep latency and help your loved one stay asleep during the night. They may not all be right for him or her, and that's perfectly okay. Select one or two that sound promising and put them into practice. After a week or so, assess how things are going and add or subtract nighttime behaviors as necessary. We hope that your loved one will find a routine that helps improve the quality of his or her sleep and yours.

1. **Develop a preferred routine.** Your loved one might decide to take a bath or a shower, wash his or her face, or brush his or her teeth every night before bed. The idea is to create a habit that the body and brain associate with sleep. As soon as he or she starts on a personal hygiene routine, the body will recognize that it's time to start shutting down for the night.

2. **Teach progressive muscle relaxation.** Progressive muscle relaxation is an easy way to relax all muscles, one set at a time. Have your loved one start by lying on his or her back in bed. Then tell him or her to tighten all the muscles in his or her feet and calves, count to three and relax them. Next, tighten and relax the muscles in the upper area of the legs (quads). Continue to tighten and relax muscle groups as you

move upwards, including the hips and buttocks, the stomach, the hands and wrists, the arms, the shoulders, the neck and the face. Don't worry if your loved one falls asleep before you've completed this exercise—many people do. Eventually your loved one will be able to practice progressive muscle relaxation without your verbal prompts if this is a method that works for him or her.

3. **Practice meditation.** There are many different kinds of meditation, but the easiest way to start is to have your loved one lie comfortably in bed and concentrate on his or her breathing. Tell your loved one to pay attention to the way each breath feels as it enters and leaves the body. If other thoughts work their way into his or her mind, tell him or her to acknowledge them briefly and then turn attention back to breathing. If this exercise is difficult for your loved one, start with small blocks of just five minutes at a time. As he or she becomes more accustomed to the procedure, work your way up to 15 to 20 minutes. Again, don't worry if he or she falls asleep while meditating—it just shows that the relaxation training is working.

4. **Spend time with pets.** If you or your loved one has pets, spending time with them can lower blood pressure, improve mood, enhance overall sense of wellbeing, and encourage relaxation before bedtime. Every household has different rules about pets in the bedroom, but many people say there is nothing quite as soothing as sleeping with a purring cat lying next to you.

5. **Gently exercise the brain.** Try doing a crossword or word search game, or play a game of Sudoku with your loved one. Encourage your loved one to continue doing the puzzle even if he or she can't solve it; the brain still learns even when you don't solve the puzzle. For those who are competitive, trying to solve a puzzle, especially one that is challenging, may not be the best method to relax before bedtime.

6. **Offer a cup of chamomile tea.** Pour the tea into your loved one's favorite cup and enjoy relaxing with a nice, warm drink together. If your loved one doesn't like chamomile tea, try decaffeinated green tea or milk instead. A word to the wise: one cup of liquid is enough—any more and frequent urination will disrupt your loved one's sleep cycle.

7. **Prepare a light snack.** It's not a good idea to go to bed hungry as hunger pangs increase sleep latency. In choosing a snack for your loved one, avoid foods with caffeine and try to get a mixture of carbohydrates, proteins and tryptophan (see Chapter 14 for sleep-promoting foods). A cup of yogurt, a peanut butter sandwich, or a small scoop of vanilla ice cream with almond slivers are all good ideas.

8. **Offer a book.** Try to avoid mysteries that can keep your loved one up all night or books with gruesome imagery that can excite the mind. Instead, consider a book of affirmations or a book of poetry depending on your loved one's preferences. He or she might also want to read from the Bible, the Torah, the Koran or any other book that is important to his or her faith. The choice of reading material should be relaxing and positive, sending him or her off to sleep in a good mood.

9. **Encourage your loved one to write in a journal.** Some people feel that writing about their days in a journal helps them discharge negative emotions. Other people use a journal to keep a gratitude list or to write down everything they have to do the next day so they don't stay awake worrying or trying to remember all their upcoming "to-dos." A journal may also be a nice keepsake with words of wisdom for your loved one to pass along to grandchildren and future generations.

10. **Play music.** Unless your loved one finds them especially relaxing, loud, upbeat and energizing tunes probably aren't the best choices. Instead, try classical music or purchase CDs with sounds of nature or guided imagery. It's best to listen to the music in another room and then have your loved one go to the bedroom when he or she starts to feel tired. As previously mentioned, an essential part of sleep hygiene is to use the bedroom only for sleep.

11. **Remind your loved one to take evening medications.** If your loved one's doctor has prescribed medications to ease the symptoms of insomnia or parasomnias, remind him or her about an hour before bedtime. Do not allow him or her to drive or engage in any risky behaviors like cooking after taking the medications because when they kick in, they tend to kick in fast. If you do not live with your loved one and are worried about him or her missing a dosage, hiring a professional caregiver to assist your loved one with a bedtime routine such as medication reminders, can help ease your mind.

12. **Prepare the bedroom for sleep.** Ideally, the bedroom should be quiet, dark, and a little cool—just what our caveman ancestors preferred. Help your loved one prepare for bed by

turning down the bed covers, turning off all the lights (unless he or she uses a nightlight for comfort or to get back and forth to the bathroom) and silencing the television, radio, CD player, or any other device that makes noise.

13. **Encourage engagement in a relaxing hobby.** If your loved one has a relaxing hobby such as needlework, painting, drawing, or woodwork, encourage him or her to spend some time doing that before bedtime. Setting aside time to do something he or she enjoys can boost mood and give him or her a sense of purpose and increased self-esteem.

14. **Help prepare for the next day.** If your loved one is the type who lies awake and worries about everything that has to be done in the morning, assist him or her in doing as much as possible the night before. For instance, you might want to help set the table for breakfast, or collect items that need to be dropped off at the post office or library and put them by the door. This is also a situation where hiring a professional caregiver may be ideal—he or she can take care of household upkeep, meal preparation and errands so your loved one has more time for socializing with friends and family and favorite activities such as gardening or painting.

15. **Have your loved one talk or write about anything that is worrying him or her.** Does your loved one have something distressing on his or her mind that makes sleeping difficult? Encourage him or her to talk about it with you, a close friend, or another trusted advisor like a religious leader. Sharing worries and concerns with someone

who cares can make the negative feelings more manageable. If your loved one doesn't feel comfortable talking about the problem, suggest that he or she write about it instead as many people find the expressive writing process itself quite cathartic.

16. **Light a candle.** People skilled in aromatherapy say that the best scents to induce relaxation include lavender, rose, sandalwood and chamomile. If none of those scents are on your loved one's "favorites" list, burn a fragrance he or she enjoys. Be sure to extinguish the candle before going to bed to avoid any potential fire hazards.

17. **Encourage your loved one to read a bedtime story to grandchildren or other younger family members.** If your loved one has grandchildren or grandnieces/grandnephews visiting, encourage the children to select one of their favorite bedtime stories to read together before bed. This will probably make your loved one tired as well. Classic bedtime stories include *Can't You Sleep, Little Bear?*, *The Quiltmaker's Gift* and *Goodnight Moon*.

18. **Create white noise.** Turn on a fan, a white noise machine, or a CD with rhythmic, soothing sounds of nature like waves crashing on a beach or a gentle spring rain splashing on the ground. These sounds can help block out other more annoying sounds such as traffic from a busy street, a party at a neighbor's house, or a partner's snoring.

19. **Dim the lights.** Remember that darkness sends signals to structures within the eyes, which then signal the brain to release melatonin. Try to make your loved one's bedroom

as dark as possible, keeping fall risk safety in mind (e.g. remove small throw rugs near the bed, ensure there are no furniture or electrical cords in the walkway, have a flashlight or night-light nearby for late-night bathroom visits).

20. **Encourage intimacy with a partner.** Intimacy doesn't just refer to sex. It could mean giving and receiving back massages or even something as simple as holding hands and whispering words of love to each other. Pleasant, intimate touch with someone you love is a mood booster and a great cure for insomnia.

21. **Encourage your loved one to use the bathroom.** Make sure your loved one's last stop before the bedroom is the bathroom. There are few things more frustrating than being almost asleep and then feeling that persistent pressure on your bladder that forces you to haul yourself out of your comfortable bed to go. As previously mentioned, getting up in the middle of the night can pose a fall risk for an aging loved one and disrupts sleep quality.

22. **Do a few stretches together.** Some people find that a few slow, gentle stretches before bedtime help them relax so that they can fall asleep more quickly. Signing up for a senior yoga or tai chi class will not only allow your loved one to socialize with peers but will also help him or her learn relaxing, flowing motions that are conducive to sleep.

23. **Set a consistent bedtime.** Humans are creatures of habit. If your loved one consistently trains his or her body to go to sleep at the same time each night, then he or she will likely find him or herself getting drowsy right on schedule for a nice, long sleep.

24. Have a mid-night wake-up procedure in place. There's nothing more counterproductive than lying awake staring at the alarm clock while minute after minute ticks away. It is best to get up for a few minutes and try one of the techniques suggested in this chapter. However, for aging loved ones who are frail or at risk for falls, getting up in the middle of the night in a dark room can be quite dangerous. Format a plan together for what to do in these cases— perhaps you can have a cell phone or walkie-talkie near the bed to facilitate communication with you or a caregiver in the home. This is another situation where hiring a professional caregiver would be ideal. He or she can stay awake through the night to assist your loved one if he or she wakes so that you can get a restful night's sleep as well.

25. Count sheep. This much-maligned method of inducing sleep actually has a lot going for it. Focusing on a simple task like counting helps to block other matters of concern from occupying the brain, and thinking about those cute little fluffy white sheep is really relaxing. See how many sheep your loved one can count the next time he or she uses this technique. Chances are, he or she won't get anywhere near 100 before falling fast asleep.

This chapter highlighted some methods your loved one can try to get a sound night's sleep. There are also, however, some behaviors that your loved one will want to avoid if the goal is rest and relaxation. The next chapter explores the 12 main activities to avoid before bedtime and explains why each one can be toxic to a restful night's sleep.

CHAPTER 18: 12 ACTIVITIES TO AVOID BEFORE BEDTIME

"Life is something that happens when you can't get to sleep."
– Fran Lebowitz

When you're trying to adopt a new habit such as good sleep hygiene, it's very important to learn what you need to do in order to reach your goal. It is equally important, however, to know what not to do. Thus, this chapter addresses 12 activities to avoid if your loved one wants to fall asleep quickly and sleep peacefully through the night.

1. **Nighttime television.** Nighttime television consists mostly of news programs with graphic footage and mystery/thriller weekly dramas, which also have some pretty explicit content. While it's great that your loved one wants to stay up to date on current affairs, the excitatory content can greatly interfere with the body's relaxation response and consequently, disrupt sleep. Instead, suggest that your loved one record his or her favorite programs and watch them in the morning or early afternoon.

2. **Eating heavy, high-fat meals.** Like nighttime television, these delightful culinary experiences are not always forbidden, but think twice before indulging just before bedtime. A heavy meal is likely to leave your loved one feeling overly full and uncomfortable as he or she tries to drift off to sleep and thus, increases sleep latency. Large, high-fat meals may also excite the brain and bring on vivid dreams or nightmares.

3. **Arguments.** The old adage, "Never go to bed angry" does hold some wisdom. For example, trying to broach the topic of care options with your resistant aging loved one at the dinner table can greatly interfere with his or her sleep quality and duration. Arguments can leave the parties involved with tense muscles, clenched jaws and even headaches or stomachaches. If an argument does occur close to bedtime, go back and work through some of the relaxing exercises in Chapter 17 with your loved one. Ideally, you can address any emotional and difficult topics in the morning or early afternoon. If your loved one has been experiencing sleep problems but is resistant to additional assistance from you, consider hiring a professional caregiver for bedtime routines. Your loved one may be more receptive to someone else coming in, making suggestions and helping with healthy sleep habits.

4. **Reading emotionally stimulating books.** Most of us have probably had the experience of picking a book up before bedtime and not putting it down again until 5:00 AM. If you've read a book like that, you've had the great luck of finding a spellbinding writer. Unfortunately, you've also found a writer who is a poor choice for bedtime reading. Encourage your loved one to save the can't-put-it-down books for the morning and afternoon. More appropriate bedtime reading materials include poetry, affirmation and prayers.

5. **Heavy exercise.** But wait a minute! Isn't exercise supposed to be good for sleep? Yes, if you time it correctly. Ever active Tanya, age 65, goes rock climbing at least twice a week and bikes for ten miles a day rain or shine. After several restless

nights, though, she noticed that if she finished her biking by mid-afternoon, she slept better. Now she winds up her bike rides by 2:00 PM, does nothing more strenuous than tai chi for the rest of the day, and sleeps like a log. Encourage your loved one to complete any aerobic exercise early in the day, transitioning to less intensive forms of exercise like tai chi or gentle yoga as the day progresses.

6. **Rough and tumble play.** As with rigorous exercise, playing tag or hide and seek with the grandkids are fine activities through the early evening hours, but if they carry on into the late evening they can leave the body feeling too amped up to sleep.

7. **Drinking caffeine.** Caffeine is found chiefly in coffee, some types of tea, soft drinks and chocolate products. As addressed in Chapter 4, the main problem with caffeine is that it takes a long time to clear out of your system. For instance, if you drink a cup of caffeinated coffee with your evening meal, about half of that caffeine will still be affecting your mood, behavior, and level of alertness when it is time for bed. If your loved one needs caffeine to jump-start his or her day, that's fine, but by mid-afternoon at the latest switch over to decaffeinated drinks.

8. **Drinking alcohol.** The most popular non-prescription central nervous system depressant is alcohol. Many people who are depressed or who can't sleep drink heavily in the evenings, hoping the alcohol will ease them into sleep. This plan often seems to work perfectly, since alcohol reduces sleep latency. As we discussed in Chapter 4, though, alcohol also disrupts the quality of sleep, preventing people from

reaching Stage 3 and Stage 4 sleep, during which most of the healing from the day's wear and tear and memory consolidation takes place (See Chapter 2). If your loved one feels that he or she can't fall asleep without help, make an appointment to see his or her doctor to discuss healthier alternatives.

9. **Taking care of business late at night.** If your loved one is busy during the day, he or she may be tempted to stay up paying bills or to take care of other household chores into the night. Doing this once in a while probably won't hurt him or her – the problem comes when late night sessions become the norm rather than the exception. The problem is even worse if your loved one is paying bills or handling other household issues from bed. Remember the golden rule of good sleep hygiene? The bed is only for sleep.

10. **Experiencing very positive or very negative emotions.** There are times when it's normal for strong positive or negative emotions to disrupt sleep. If a loved one passed away recently, for instance, or if your mom just found out she is going to be a grandmother, lying awake pondering feelings and changes for a night or two would not be terribly worrisome. Strong emotions only become a problem when they become a pattern. For instance, if your loved one seems to be living on a high almost every day and feels as if he or she doesn't need sleep, he or she may be having a manic episode or a reaction to a medication and you will want to visit the doctor as soon as possible. Your loved one should also visit a physician if she or he is persistently feeling sad and pessimistic and if these negative thoughts are keeping him or her awake.

11. **Ruminating about problems.** Ruminating means to continuously, even compulsively, focus attention on past negative experiences or feelings. Ruminating isn't an attempt to gain greater insight or understand the source of problem, but rather an excessive rehashing of anxiety-provoking thoughts and beliefs. In fact, people who ruminate dwell on the same problem without making progress in understanding their feelings. Those who ruminate respond very well to cognitive behavioral therapy, which challenges the person to come up with more positive and realistic outcomes. ("My landlord threatened to kick me out if I miss another monthly payment; I'll call my children and ask if they can remind me every month so I don't accidentally forget.")

12. **Interruptions.** If your loved one shares a home with you or other family members, you will probably interrupt his or her sleep once in a while. Some interruptions are valid, like a sick child or a household emergency. Others, though, are merely inconsiderate. Be careful not to let those occasional inconsiderate interruptions become a habit. Tell your family that when your senior loved one goes into the bedroom and closes the door at night, you don't want him or her to be disturbed absent of a true crisis. If the people who live with you feel compelled to test that edict (and they will), practice saying no. For example, say "Grandma will play checkers with you tomorrow. This is her sleeping time."

This concludes the last chapter of our book. We hope that you have learned the mechanisms behind what happens during sleep and why getting at least seven to nine hours of sleep each night is so important for the body. If your senior loved one has been experiencing sleep issues, we hope this guide has provided some insight into what may be preventing quality sleep and how you can work with your loved one and his or her physician to overcome these barriers. Most important, we hope that you have taken away the key point that sleep problems are not a normal part of aging and there is a spectrum of behaviors and interventions that can improve sleep and thus quality of life at any age.

If you're taking care of a senior citizen, or if you know someone else who is, you might want to read Appendix A, which discusses sleep problems caregivers deal with and how to resolve them.

We also hope you'll spend some time looking through Appendix B, which includes various resources to help you keep your own sleep—and your elderly loved one's sleep—on track.

APPENDIX A: SLEEP FOR THE CAREGIVER

"One person caring about another represents life's greatest value."
– Jim Rohn

When it became clear that Gina's widowed father, Arthur, was experiencing some serious cognitive problems, she decided to move in with him. She and her dad had always gotten along well and she did not anticipate that caring for him would be difficult. She hired a caregiver to help Art during the week while she worked and she took over care on the nights and weekends.

No one had warned Gina about sundowning, a term used to describe symptoms of agitation and confusion in the evening and nighttime hours, common in those in the middle stages of Alzheimer's. Gina also didn't know that Art hadn't slept well in years. Many times she stayed up most of the night with her restless father, catching only an hour or two of sleep herself before drowsily driving to her office for another grueling day of work.

Gina is not alone. Many caregivers struggle to get the sleep they need while caring for an aging loved one. Having to physically assist a loved one during the night is one of many factors that can disrupt a caregiver's sleep cycle. Lack of sleep can initiate and/or heighten some of the most common emotions associated with caregiving and these emotions can further disrupt the sleep cycle.

Worry and Stress

One night, about three months after Gina moved in with her father, she was so exhausted she fell asleep on the couch for a few minutes. During that time, Art managed to wander out the back door. The police found him several blocks from his home and brought him back to Gina. They gave her a stern warning about the importance of supervising Art. She felt horribly guilty. From that night on, even if she waited until Art was deeply asleep before she went to bed, she tossed and turned, worrying that he would wander out of the house again.

If you're a caregiver, you may spend time worrying about your loved one—how you can protect her from harm, what you will do when his condition worsens, how to do the best job you possibly can while still meeting commitments to other people in your life. Worry is one of many factors that can keep you from getting a restful night's sleep.

Anticipatory Grieving

Gina had only been living with Art for about a month, and she could see his health and his cognitive abilities declining before her eyes. One evening over dinner he looked across the table and asked her, "Do I have any children?" Gina, an only child and once the apple of her father's eye, was devastated.

When you learn that a loved one has a life-limiting illness, it's normal to start grieving for him or for her before death actually occurs. You may miss the things the two of you used to be able to do together or you may grieve for the cognitive abilities your loved one has lost. This sadness and grief is natural, but grief can disrupt the sleep cycle, making it difficult to fall asleep and to stay asleep. Gina often cried herself to sleep at night, wishing her father would come to comfort her as he had when she was a child and had nightmares.

Loneliness/Isolation

Gina had a large circle of friends and several aunts, uncles, and cousins. She never expected to be lonely, but as Art's declines became more noticeable, people stopped coming by and rarely called. "I'm sure you and Art have a routine set up," one of Gina's aunts said. "I wouldn't dream of interrupting your day." Others were more forthright. "I'm sorry, Gina," one friend said, "but I just can't bear to see your father that way."

There are several reasons why caregivers become isolated. Sometimes the people they counted on for support are simply not up to the task. They may be afraid to face the realities of a serious medical condition, or they may not know what to say or how to act around the person who is ill.

Sometimes, however, it is the caregiver who backs away from others. He or she may feel, for instance, that nobody could possibly understand what he or she is going through, or it may be easier to function as a caregiver without being around friends and the memories of happier times.

Finally, you may find that with your caregiving schedule you don't have time to get together with friends or family members. Even taking an evening off for dinner and a movie means having to find a surrogate caregiver, and this can be a daunting task.

While loneliness alone probably won't rob you of sleep, the feeling of isolation and lack of emotional support associated with loneliness can contribute to depression. And depression can lead to problems falling and staying asleep.

While a few nights of tossing and turning usually don't have serious consequences, long-term sleep deprivation can result in errors in judgment, poor performance on the job or as a caregiver, accidents caused by sleepiness and an overall lower quality of life. Gina not only started to make more mistakes at work, she was also involved in a couple of fender benders caused by her inability to concentrate while driving.

Fatigue

After six months, Gina had had it. She could hardly stay awake during the day and sleep refused to come at night. She often locked herself in the bathroom and cried. She began to think about something she'd often said she would never consider—putting Art in an assisted living facility.

Many caregivers experience fatigue, and some make care decisions for their loved ones based on that fatigue.

Finding Help

Making up your sleep debt can give you a whole new perspective on planning your loved one's care. In order to do this, though, you may have to commit to making some major changes. That may mean reaching out to family members—even those who have backed away—and telling them that you can no longer manage your loved one's care alone. Ask specifically for what you need. For instance, you might say, "I need you to take Dad for the weekends so I can get some rest," or "I need money to help hire a private duty caregiver." If the first people you ask can't help you, keep asking.

Family members who are squeamish about handling personal care may be more than willing to help you out financially. Use those funds to hire a caregiver for as many hours as you can afford. Home Care Assistance is one source of highly-trained and experienced caregivers that provide exceptional care to clients throughout North America (see Appendix B for contact information).

You probably won't sleep the first time someone comes by to provide respite care to your loved one. That's normal. You may want to watch your loved one interact with the caregiver for some time before you leave them alone. Once you are at ease, do something relaxing—take a bubble bath, read a book, have dinner out with a friend. After a few visits, you may feel comfortable lying down for a nap while the caregiver visits with your loved one.

Another option is to hire a nighttime caregiver for your loved one. This will allow you the chance to catch up on sleep without having to worry about your loved one wandering out of the house or accidentally injuring him or herself.

If you've had insomnia for several weeks or months, you may find that it's difficult to get back into a regular sleep schedule. Talk to your doctor. He or she may recommend a hypnotic medication like zolpidem or a mild sedative. He or she may also suggest that you talk to a mental health professional or a member of the clergy to get extra emotional support and to talk through options about your loved one's care.

Other Options

For many families, money is tight and affording care for your loved one may be difficult. Check and see if your loved one has a long-term care insurance policy. These policies often cover the cost of care in the home as well as in a nursing home.

Another idea is to call your local hospital and ask to speak to the social services department. They can help you find care options for which your loved one may be eligible. Depending on your loved one's current physical condition and mental state, options will vary anywhere from in-home care to moving him or her to a facility to hospice care. There may also be community agencies that provide volunteers for respite service. If you or your loved one is affiliated with a local church, talk to the pastor and see if there are any church members who are willing to donate a few hours a week to care for your loved one. If your loved one is a veteran, see if you can get him or her involved in programs at the local VA.

After you think about all your options, you may decide that the most appropriate place for your loved one to receive care is a skilled nursing facility. That's a perfectly reasonable choice. Many people thrive in a nursing home setting.

Whatever your decision, however, it should be made with careful thought and clarity, and not in a haze of sleep-deprivation. Get some extra help, catch up on your sleep and make a rational, informed choice about what is good for you, as well as for your loved one.

Gina, for instance, called all of Art's siblings together for a family meeting and told them about Art's sundowning and her own difficulty providing care for him. Since all of Gina's aunts and uncles were senior citizens themselves, none felt qualified to care for Art when he was restless at night. The family did, however, chip in with enough money for Gina to hire a professional caregiver from a private duty company five nights a week.

The first week was difficult. It took Art some time to get used to a new person in the house, and he "fired" his caregiver regularly. Gina was sure that this plan would turn out to be a dead end.

The caregiver, however, was patient and gentle, and by the second week, Art had gotten used to having her around. He still had his days and nights confused, but when he got up and wandered, the caregiver watched him so Gina could sleep.

During the next few months, the caregiver gave Gina advice on daytime activities and different foods that might help Art sleep better at night. He never entirely returned to a normal sleep schedule, but he did fall asleep more quickly and stay asleep longer than he had in the past.

The arrangement continued for almost a year, until Art died peacefully in his sleep.

He passed away in his home, just as he had always wanted. Gina, no longer sleep-deprived, took a leave of absence from work and spent their last days together providing physical care for her father, telling him about her memories of her happy childhood and the wonderful relationship they had shared, or simply holding his hand and sitting quietly at his side.

After Art died, she could honestly say that she had no regrets.

Unlike many long-term caregivers, she was also in relatively good health herself. Hiring a professional caregiver allowed her the time to pursue her own interests, catch up on sleep and make sure that her own physical, emotional and spiritual needs were met.

Caring for a loved one with a sleep disorder is probably one of the most difficult things you will ever do. Please don't feel as if you have to go through it alone. Having a professional caregiver on board can make all the difference in the world, both to your loved one's health and to your own.

If you've been putting off making that call for help, get on the phone and do it now. You won't be sorry.

APPENDIX B: RESOURCES

"A well-spent day brings happy sleep." – Leonardo da Vinci

Books about Sleep, Dreams and Sleep Disorders

The Cleveland Guide to Sleep Disorders, by Nancy Foldvary-Schaefer (Kaplan Publishing, 2009).

The Harvard Medical School's Guide to a Good Night's Sleep, by Lawrence Epstein and Steven Mardon (McGraw-Hill, 2006).

The Insomnia Workbook: A Comprehensive Guide to Getting You the Sleep You Need, by Stephanie Silberman (New Harbinger Publications, 2009).

Master Your Sleep – Proven Methods Simplified, by Tracey I. Marks (Bascom Hill Publishing Group, 2011).

The Mind at Night: The New Science of How and Why We Dream, by Andrea Rock (Basic Books, 2005).

The Post-Traumatic Insomniac Workbook: A Step-by-Step Program for Overcoming Sleep Problems after Trauma, by Karin Elorriaga Thompson and C. Laurel Franklin (New Harbinger Publications, 2010).

The Promise of Sleep: A Pioneer in Sleep Medicine Explores the Vital Connection Between Health, Happiness, and a Good Night's Sleep, by William C. Dement (Dell, 2000).

Restful Insomnia: How to Get the Benefits of Sleep Even When you Can't, by Sondra Kornblatt (Conari Press, 2010).

Sleep: A Groundbreaking Guide to the Mysteries, the Problems, and the Solutions, by Carlos H. Schenck (Avery Trade, 2008).

Read Your Loved One to Sleep at Night

20-Minute Retreats: Revive Your Spirit in Just Minutes a Day with Simple, Self-Led Practices, by Rachel Harris (Holt Paperbacks, 2000).

Chicken Soup for the Soul: Think Positive: 101 Inspirational Stories about Counting Your Blessings and Having a Positive Attitude, by Jack Canfield, Mark Victor Hansen, and Amy Newmark (Chicken Soup for the Soul, 2010).

Couple's Comfort Book: A Creative Guide for Renewing Passion, Pleasure, and Commitment, by Jennifer Louden (HarperOne, 2005).

The Wealthy Spirit: Daily Affirmations for Financial Stress Reduction, by Chellie Campbell (Sourcebooks, 2002).

Woman's Comfort Book: A Self-Nurturing Guide for Restoring Balance in Your Life, by Jennifer Louden (HarperOne, reprint 2005).

Bedtime Stories – Can be very soothing to people with advanced dementia

Can't You Sleep, Little Bear? by Martin Waddell and Barbara Firth (Candlewick, 1995).

Dr. Seuss's Sleep Book, by Dr. Seuss (Random House Books for Young Readers, 1962).

Goodnight, Little Bear, by Richard Scarry (Golden Books, 2001).

Goodnight Moon Classic Library: Contains Goodnight Moon, the Runaway Bunny, and My World, by Margaret Wise Brown and Clement Hurd (HarperCollins, 2011).

The Quiltmaker's Gift, by Jeff Brumbeau and Gail de Marcken (Scholastic Press, 3rd edition 2001).

You Are Special (Max Lucado's Wemmicks), by Max Lucado and Sergio Martinez (Crossway, 1997).

CDs to Encourage Relaxation and Sleep

Deep Sleep Every Night, by Glenn Harrold (Diviniti Publishing, 2002).

Deep Sleep with Medical Self-Hypnosis, by Steven Gurgevich (Sounds True Incorporated, 2009).

Health Journeys: A Meditation to Help You with Healthful Sleep, by Belleruth Naparstek (Health Journeys, 2000).

Hypnosis to Help You Sleep Deeply, by Janet I. Decker (Hypnotherapy Services, 2007)

Sleep Through Insomnia: Meditations to Quiet the Mind and Still the Body, by KRS Edstrom (Soft Stone Publishing, 2005).

Sound Sleep: Relax for Deep Sleep, by Kelly Howell (Brain Sync, 2001).

Helpful Websites

Sleep/Dreams/Sleep Disorders
American Sleep Association
http://www.sleepassociation.org/index.php

The Bruxism Association
http://www.bruxism.org.uk

HelpGuide.org – Insomnia
http://www.helpguide.org/life/insomnia_treatment.htm

Insomnialand – Genuine Insomnia Help
http://www.insomnialand.com

International Association for the Study of Dreams
http://asdreams.org/index_pre_2013.htm

NAMI – National Alliance on Mental Illness
http://www.nami.org

National Sleep Foundation
http://www.sleepfoundation.org

The Sleep Well
http://www.stanford.edu/~dement

Senior Care
AGIS – Assist Guide Information Services: Articles and Education about Sleep Issues
http://www.agis.com/Search/Search.aspx?type=doc&q=Sleep+Issues

Alzheimer's Association: Sleep Issues and Sundowning
http://www.alz.org/care/alzheimers-dementia-sleep-issues-sundowning.asp

OUR MISSION

Our mission at Home Care Assistance is to change the way the world ages. We provide older adults with quality care that enables them to live happier, healthier lives at home. Our services are distinguished by the caliber of our caregivers, the responsiveness of our staff and our expertise in Live-In care. We embrace a positive, balanced approach to aging centered on the evolving needs of older adults.

- Live-In Experts. We specialize in around the clock care to help seniors live well at home.

- Available 24/7. Care managers are on call for clients and their families, even during nights and weekends.

- High Caliber Caregivers. We hire only 1 in 25 applicants and provide ongoing training and supervision.

- Balanced Care. Our unique approach to care promotes healthy mind, body and spirit.

- No Long Term Contracts. Use our services only as long as you're 100% satisfied.

- A Trusted Partner. We're honored to be Preferred Providers for professionals in both the medical and senior communities.

- Peace of Mind. Independent industry surveys place our client satisfaction rate at 97%.

AUTHOR BIOGRAPHIES

Kathy N. Johnson, PhD, CMC is a Certified Geriatric Care Manager and Chief Executive Officer of Home Care Assistance. A recognized leader in senior care, she holds a Doctorate in Psychology from the Illinois Institute of Technology.

James H. Johnson, PhD is a licensed clinical psychologist and Chairman of Home Care Assistance. He is the former department chair of the Virginia Consortium for Professional Psychology and the award-winning author of nine books. He holds a Doctorate in Psychology from the University of Minnesota.

Lily Sarafan, MS is President and Chief Operating Officer of Home Care Assistance. She has been featured as an industry expert by more than 100 media outlets. She holds Masters and Bachelors degrees from Stanford University.

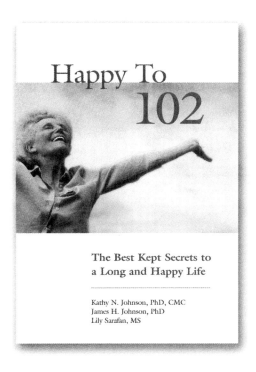

Available on amazon.com.

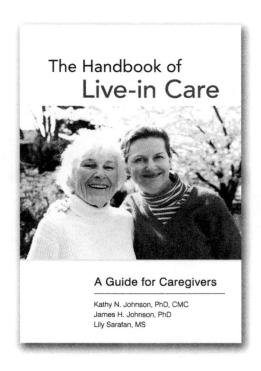

Available on amazon.com.

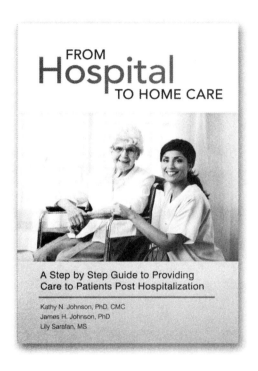

Available on **amazon**.COM.

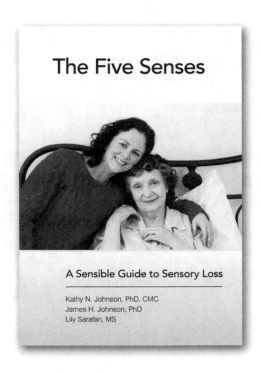

Available on amazon.com.

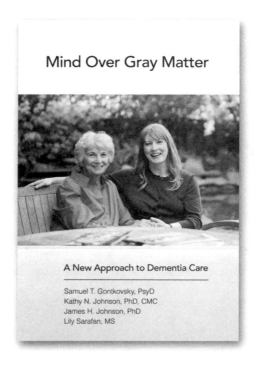

Available on **amazon**.com.

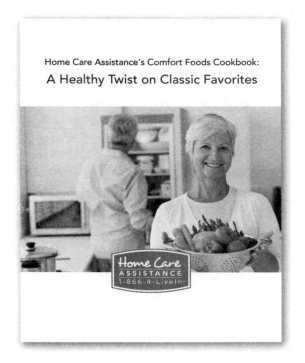